Trans Femme Futures

'Astute and hopeful, *Trans Femme Futures* manages to divulge profound theoretical insights of trans liberation as intimate and soulful endeavours of trans living and world making on the margins. Offering up an abolitionist "transfeminist love-politics" as a practical antidote to the suffocating neoliberal world order, the book is a breath of fresh air amidst stale and moribund, if long rehearsed, existing bad faith discourses on gender and its many troubles.'

—H.L.T. Quan, author of *Become Ungovernable*

'A brilliant, useful, and immensely moving book that deals a critical blow to the epistemic austerity of our times. With their chromatic defence of theory as a "tool to work upon the imagination", Nat Raha and Mijke van der Drift have exemplified that rare and precious genre of revolutionary writing that knows how to buoy and calm its reader enough to absorb complex argument and body forward its stakes.'

—Jordy Rosenberg, author of *Confessions of the Fox*

'A radical and sensuous ethics of trans femme complicity, collectivity and worldmaking, Raha and van der Drift theorise anti-colonial femmes practices which "undo the grip of empire on the soul through the senses" in this beautiful and necessary work.'

—Trish Salah, Associate Professor of Gender Studies, Queen's University and author of *Wanting in Arabic*

'When one thinks of trans, feminism, and radical as genuinely, inextricably entangled, one thinks of this book. This is what we need at this moment: a powerful, steadfast commitment to liberation. And this is it.'

—Marquis Bey, author of *Black Trans Feminism*

'A theoretically rich account of the forms of care that support the well-being of transfeminine people, showing how these caring practices link up tangibly to what could be called an ethics of abolition.'

—Mattie Armstrong-Price, Assistant Professor of History, Fordham University

Trans Femme Futures

Abolitionist Ethics for Transfeminist Worlds

Nat Raha and Mijke van der Drift

First published 2024 by Pluto Press
New Wing, Somerset House, Strand, London WC2R 1LA
and Pluto Press, Inc.
1930 Village Center Circle, 3-834, Las Vegas, NV 89134

www.plutobooks.com

British Library Cataloguing in Publication Data
A catalogue record for this book is available from the British Library

ISBN 978 0 7453 4940 4   Paperback
ISBN 978 0 7453 4942 8   PDF
ISBN 978 0 7453 4941 1   EPUB

This book is printed on paper suitable for recycling and made from fully
managed and sustained forest sources. Logging, pulping and manufacturing
processes are expected to conform to the environmental standards of the
country of origin.

Typeset by Stanford DTP Services, Northampton, England

Simultaneously printed in the United Kingdom and United States of America

Contents

Introduction
Trans liberation is between us

Trans liberation is a collective movement to free all people from regimes of gender oppression through social and material transformation. Trans lives have transgressed and challenged these regimes through changing or refusing gender, which we propose is a collective effort that emerges through the practices we undertake together. In *Trans Femme Futures* we focus on the fabric of trans, queer, feminist, and abolitionist living and world-making, and of trans femme lives in particular, to consider how our lives are shaped by sensuous and collective movements. We detail the importance of practices that transform our everyday lives – such as practising solidarity, support, care, theorising and embodied transformation – in the dismantling of forms of duress faced by trans, non-binary, gender non-conforming, and queer people (especially in the context of other intermeshing marginalisations). In this, this book intends to shift trans, queer, feminist, and anti-racist dialogues, and understandings of oppression away from identity by emphasising the importance of what we do, and how and why we do it, towards the (re)making of our lives, together.

TRANSFEMINISM, ETHICS, AND COLLECTIVES

We describe collective making of forms of life as *ethics*, which is the way futures manifest – through building and maintaining the worlds and ways of living that enable our existences and our thriving. We choose the term ethics, in contrast to the spaces of politics, rights, and norms which endeavour to counter, break or assimilate trans life. Trans life entails actively embodying social change, opting for paths along which one may flourish, even if that means facing harm and challenges. Trans proposes a movement away – an escape – from imposed categories or starting points,[1] which shows trans as creative and collective acts. Transness doesn't strive for a pre-determined outcome, but takes shape along the way – sensually and relationally. Countering the idea that the good life is defined by normative consensus, material wealth, and purchasing power, we find it in nourishing, interconnected and interdependent relationships with other humans and non-human life and in the space for differences to develop without losing connection. We use ethics to address the commonalities amid different forms of flourishing and working together, and care for mutual differences. Trans life entails embracing the possibilities of embodied, social and soulful approaches to the world, possibilities that may bring joy.

For us, transfeminism entails deep study of the relational skills and knowledges that exist between us. Our intention is to elaborate on the possibilities of transfeminism beyond a politics encumbered with contesting people who think trans people should not – or do not – exist. Against currents that work to reinforce structural transphobia and everyday violence against trans people, we consider what emerges when our idea of political struggle is not centred on the liberal political arena and rights, nor the media. Our transfeminist ethics is not defined by forms that cohere through institutions, even if, as we discuss throughout the book, trans life is repeatedly encumbered by institutions. Institutions suggest that the pressures upon trans lives may be solved by inclusion. Abolitionist approaches, by contrast, help us understand why inclusion is conditional and how we can navigate institutions should we need to, while advocating for other possibilities. These approaches also require that we think through questions of complicity regarding institutions and the harmful dynamics born out of social hierarchies, reconsidering our agency in their midst.

This book centres femmeness through trans, and trans through femmeness – a reclaimed, queer, politicised, and sensuous understanding and practice of femininity. Femmeness is about the stakes of putting oneself out there, of nurturing each other and oneself, knowing that one is an agent of pleasure and possibility in one's life – even in a world that is willing to use, exploit or destroy you. Feminism encourages us to learn from the forms of harm and violence that emerge within hetero- and cis-normative, ableist, racial patriarchal capitalism and the structures that enable it. The legacies of anti-colonial and anti-capitalist, feminist resistance show multiple ways that we can build alternatives together. We propose that trans femme flourishing emerges from abolition, as abolition undoes structures of repression that enable the violence faced by trans femmes. Even when this violence is not direct, it is present in the affects and emotions inscribed through trans bodies. The threat of punishment for not falling into line with norms is an element of patriarchal institutionalism. Violence – locking people out, enclosing people in – is the normative method of wrestling control. Abolition is the opposite, and to address frictions, tensions, and crises without recourse to violence, we need collectivity and community. For H.L.T. Quan, mass movements are a space for friendship, on the road to abolition of violent institutions.[2]

The idea of a singular, unified, and identifiable 'trans community' (or 'LGBT+ community') is regularly hailed in the service of queer and trans liberalism and other neoliberal political endeavours, but it typically is a misnomer for trans, non-binary and gender non-conforming people that fails to understand us. The idea that all members of a community share a commonality of experience (for example, that trans people gather around an experience of disconnect from the gender we were assigned at birth) tends to flatten out important nuances and differences between us (for instance, that gender deviance is policed differently according to different codes of race, class, and positioning).[3] In contrast to neoliberal approaches, collective ones can provide a space to practice and develop actions and skills, modes of expression and desire, informing the direction of our aims while attending to our needs.

THEORY FOR LIBERATION

While thinking through social and collective practices, this book grounds transfeminism in theory. Theory has a role in the transformation of the world. We write in a time of fabricated scarcity, visibly economic but also epistemic (relating to knowledge), relegating theory to a much more limited and disembodied form than that which we need for transformation and liberation. Theory intermingles with how we engage with the world and each other, of how we come together, how we know, what we know, and how we think. Theory can build bridges across provincialised thought by remaining connected to other ways of living, thinking, and relating. While the local is important for the grounding of understanding, it can demand a sameness that is suffocating. Constellating insights across different localities provides tools and modes of thought, letting theory expand the local because it is a tool to work upon the imagination itself. And in that manner, theory works against patriarchy.

Anti-colonial thought and critical European philosophies underline how imperial norms rely heavily on generalised and abstract thought.[4] Hegemonic generalisations encompass and traverse a range of contexts to enable long-distance control, as Anibal Quijano explains, while the coloniality of power relies on the institutionalisation of life.[5] Institutionalisation creates indifference and encourages a contraction of perception through generalisations: if groups behave 'the same', relations are pre-figured. Michel Foucault and Immanuel Kant claim that experience and generalisations are of the same logical form – for instance, in Foucault's understanding the convict thinks of 'himself' only as prisoner, because the hegemonic image is omnipresent.[6] This idea is echoed in contemporary pigeon-holing through identity categories, both in how one is perceived by other people or institutions, and how one may conceive of oneself, and what is possible in one's life. However, María Lugones, Denise Ferreira da Silva, and many others help us see how abstractions are necessary to understand contexts. We need abstractions, because pattern recognition relies on it.[7] Escaping a normative environment relies in part on theory – liberation involves both experience and pattern recognition. The replacement of relationality with generalities, in the form of norms, policy and generic identity categories, beckons us away from the link between the sensuous and the abstract, which holds the potential for new forms of living. Thus, we make a strong case for theory and analytical approaches that are scaled up from immediate bodily being.

This book is written in a variety of voices and styles. From the deeply embodied to the analytical, the book speaks in different registers. As a book on abolitionist ethics, its voice is embodied, because ethics is action combined with thought. Mixing personal, theoretical, and embodied styles, we aim to show that a multiplicity of voices can speak a more complete truth.

We are living in a time that seems to be post-social consensus, post-welfare state, post-critique, post-truth and post-Tumblr; meanwhile, it remains a challenge to recognise how capitalism and nation-states co-opt social movement struggles. The mounting pressure on trans lives in the last few years has shown us that information spreads along social fault lines, even if people generally know much more about trans life than 15 years ago. Rampant urban gentrification deprives us of collective social spaces for the exploration of possibility. This scarcity reflects the austerity of a Global North, European context in which we write, in which publics are told that there is no money or space (or jobs) despite over 500 years of global colonial extraction, dispossession, exploitation, and accumulation that has enriched Europe. Theory is one way to make up for the loss of social and embodied space. It is not a replacement of other social spaces, but an addition to them. We need tools to reflect and reimagine how we will build and make our lives without recourse to systems that don't serve us, nor the majority of people on this planet. Caught between the falsity of the promise of inclusion and the reality of disposability, between medical violence and niche possibilities, flourishing requires thought about actions and activities, rather than prioritising knowledge and understanding. Flourishing requires possibilities for conversation and political imagination, but more importantly, to highlight how we can relate to each other.

Social movements nonetheless continue to put the promise of liberation into practice. The Black Lives Matter movement has put contemporary racist and anti-Black structures firmly on the agenda, and put proposals and practices to abolish the police into the mainstream. At the time of writing, we are witnessing and participating in the largest social movement of this generation – the movement for, and in solidarity with, the liberation of Palestine. States and institutions are showing their true colours in the support of military might, settler colonialism, apartheid and genocide – over the protection of Palestinian lives. Yet as the war in Gaza rages on, we see the dynamics of a growing social movement and the relationships that are forged. The movement spreads knowledge about the historical dispossession and struggles, the culture and lives of the Palestinian people; and knowledge is created in encampments, marches, blockades, and organising for boycotts, divestment, and sanctions. International law, coming into force through the International Court of Justice and International Criminal Court rulings on the plausibility of genocide, are unable to block the ongoing violence against Palestinians, which underlines for us: abolition is anti-colonial, anti-military, and anti-border.

The chapters of this book interweave the dynamics of collectivity, institutional critique, and proposals for liberatory action. In Chapter 1, we ground femmeness in collective contexts, to propose how the work of solidarity structures shared queer and trans femme lives. We look at collectives through our complicity in different practices, to question how our actions close worlds and open them. Chapter 2 centres care as key to transfeminist ethics. We consider how social worlds are made and unmade, focusing upon the different approaches to community. We use the concept of affective economies to address social dynamics that render trans lives disposable, attending to gendered forms of harm.

In Chapter 3 we return to the idea of complicity to consider our connections to institutions, social hierarchies, and managerialisms, and how these can filter into collective worlds. We discuss calls for trans rights and the limits of liberal trans politics, questioning the push for social inclusion amid the wider dynamics of division and separation in contemporary Europe – of the 'Hostile Environment', borders, racism, and xenophobia.

Chapter 4 focuses on medical institutions and the dire state of trans healthcare, including the violence of racial and gendered norms that structure these contexts. We discuss challenges in accessing trans-specific healthcare and the problem of psychiatric power over trans bodyminds. We propose Liberatory Harm Reduction as framework for collective practices, rather than relying on an individualised autonomy, which, we argue, fails to counter the unequal power dynamics of the Gender Clinic.

We end the book by proposing ways to bring futures into the present. We discuss solidarity as a practice infused with an ethics of generosity, one that emphasises collectivity over being right. It is through an expansive approach to solidarity that collectives can thrive while being open to the world.

1

'They would plant the rose garden themselves'

Femme, complicity, and the rewiring of the sensuous[1]

Within the currents of patriarchal, racial capitalism, femininity is caught within exploitative and gendered norms. Those of us who express and embody femininity are readily accused of conforming to socially regressive, patriarchal ideals, such as grounding our self-expression in consumption. Next to this, we are expected to undertake care and other forms of social reproductive labour on demand.[2] Whether one is trans or not, Brown or Black or white, we are confronted by these gendered pressures and norms. There is a multitude of practical responses to such expectations, from separatism to conformity, refusal to claim one is innocent, to working through one's ambivalence, and outright rebellion. By upending and playing with gender(ed) norms, femmes engage in everyday analysis of gendered dynamics and tropes, proliferating modes of trans and queer femininity.[3]

As we set out in this book, this happens in the midst of social and political relations, which cross-pollinate ideas and practices of queer and trans femininity. Throughout the book, we discuss how – in the face of duress – solidarity, friendship, political actions, and creativity between queer and trans femmes and folks more broadly create spaces for openness and becoming. We understand this as world-making or worlding. In a world different senses of meaning, history, people, narratives, and insights are brought together. A world doesn't need to be complete, but it is lived and shared.[4] With

8

such practices in mind, we theorise femme as anti-institutional and as embodied institutional critique.

Furthermore, white femininity and feminism often relies on tropes of innocence and neutrality to maintain relationships with institutions – even those that work to contain feminism's transformative potential. However, by bringing femmeness into dialogue with abolitionist thinking, we propose an ethics that embraces complicity instead. This ethics centres sociality as a mode of self-understanding that guides one's actions, uprooting (neo)liberal attitudes that try to evade friction by doling out punishment and exclusion. Instead of reforming the structures of oppression, femme encourages us to unlearn and uproot demands that reproduce social and material oppressions, to open ourselves up to social and sensorial transformation, and to take agency over the (re)construction and nourishment of our own worlds – to plant the rose garden of struggle for liberation ourselves.

CHANGING FEMME

In the meeting between trans and femme – the movement from a presupposed or assigned position within the gender binary towards something else; and a sexual identity that understands femininity as a source of power and agency – femme draws elements of femininity out of the gravitational field of racialised gender norms, severing them from their overdetermination within the gender binary and compulsory heteronormativity. This includes conceptualising, understanding, and practising femininity without it appearing as the polar opposite of masculinity. Indeed, queer femmes pick up and put into play elements stereotypically associated with both femininity and masculinity, sometimes laughingly framing this practice as being 'a bad femme'. This occurs within contexts where both normative and transgressive expressions of gender are always already encoded through hierarchies of racialisation – where whiteness frames the forms of masculinity and femininity that are socially valued and desirable (forms which are also accessible to trans people, and not just to cisgender people, even if these forms also align with cisnormativity). Femmes recast elements of femininity, combining elements of our deep desires, to a sense of how we want to be in the world, to how we wish to move through and transform it. These elements may be aligned to cultural and subcultural images; and herstories and hirstories of desire; self-expression and coming together; with formative relationships in our upbringing – what we have seen in family members and friends, adults, aunts, and siblings in other contexts – elements that have animated our sense of self-expression and possibility. Femmes shape different socialities that give form to worlds they want to live in. Our socialities burgeon from resistance, reclamation, and celebration, taking forms that draw impurely from the possibilities of nonnormativity. Above all, we argue that to be attenuated to new forms invites curiosity, openness, and a willingness to face frictions. Social change is never homogenous or emerging from a single model, but from a proliferation of forms that come together, fall apart, and invite lived reflection. Becoming is not abstract, but active and practical, and we come to know ourselves with the aid of others.

We write of femme from the particulars of our ensouled bodies, where bodily change has influenced our philosophy and our everyday practices of life, and influenced the lives and worlds we have shared with other femmes, trans people, and queers. But let us be clear from the outset: we understand femme as a practice, or way of life, that is necessarily open to sociality, regardless of gender. Femme in our formulation holds openness to change as a core element. Furthermore, we wish to dissolve a reductive idea of a singular trans femme body – *a* body that is legibly and visibly trans, in public or in private. Trans femme embodiments exist in a vast multiplicity – inflected by race, ability, sexuality, size, health, and access to healthcare. These elements, alongside our experiences, are all woven into our flesh, elements we carry into our constitution. In a world where transsexuality is primarily medicalised, access to hormones, surgeries and other treatments appear to be the most defining factors for trans embodiment; and while access to healthcare obviously influences one's bodily being, this alone does not define trans femininity. To succumb our bodily being to healthcare is to sacrifice our agency to medicine, and to its manifestations as medical industrial complex and administrative violence. (We focus our attention on healthcare in Chapter 4.) Our bodies are shaped by our labour, by our education, and much more.

We find focal points for our agency in books, TV shows, films, music, and conversations, in our networks of care and our modes of survival. (We discuss care in detail in Chapter 2.) The labour conditions which curb, allow, or demand gendered expression, the education that determines forms of expression and makes demands on our activity and mental states, influence our bodies too.[5] By stating that social change is embodied, we claim our ensouled bodyminds as contextual, and sociality as the mode we draw on to navigate our surroundings.[6] Our context is rarely singular, not only shifting between formal and informal zones of relationality, but also international contexts, and intellectual contexts that shift with sociality. Knowledge is fluid and means different things in different contexts. Becoming is not 'rooted' in a single self-centred subjectivity – the modernist appeal for self-knowledge as knowledge about one's place in the world – but it is a practical process, in relation, that relies on contextual arrangements to learn what needs to be known – knowing ourselves to be many, in many different worlds. To thrive in plurality, we embrace curiosity and generosity, to ourselves and to others. In Chapter 5 we offer a deeper discussion on generosity as ethics.

In describing queer, trans femininity as a site of creating power, we locate an aesthetics of gendering within queer and trans social life, and more specifically within subcultures. Such aesthetics can be points of contact and invitation. Subcultural femininities find their roots in a veritable mix of working-class queer bar cultures, Black and Brown ballroom cultures, minoritised ethnic cultures that have relocated and creolised, punk and goth subcultures, fandom focused on anime, graphic arts and illustration, queer perversions, and readings of Bollywood and adjacent cinemas (to identify a few). These subcultural contexts mix cultural production and performance, appropriating capital-intensive commodified culture, to bring together visual and cultural aesthetics to enact transformations, dreams and desires of gender. This creates expressions, experimentations and encodings of femininity that constellate socialities. Across such different contexts, we hold and share space for emotions (from the joyous to the difficult), creating opportunities to share skills, inspire looks, and fantasies, to dress up and glimmer.

How femme emerges through these contexts is also inflected by the site and location of these often dispersed subcultures and where one finds herself. A mix of geography, herstory/hirstory, and the dynamics of racial capitalism, modulates what aesthetics of femme appear possible in a certain location. Hirstory here may mirror the hi(r)storical moment we find ourselves within, and the presence or traces of femmes who have come before: who organised parties, made zines or sex toys, or deejayed; or started a discussion group or survivor meeting group or a book co-operative or independent press; or shared hormones with other trans folks; or taught other queers to sew, fix roofs, bake vegan goods and make roti, or any number of other things or all of them over time, and thus transformed worlds and particular spaces. The influence of the racial and gendered division of labour within queer and trans subcultures, and expectations about femmes, may shape some of these acts. And yet, to make a difference in the fabrication of queer worlds enhances the very possibility of gender's fabrication. Femme work speaks to the possibilities of one's world. If Black and Brown, migrant, crip and Mad, and non-binary people and trans femmes are making art in your vicinity, the visions of how one might create and feel through their own forms of expression, clothe themselves and assemble one's face with colour, forge a sense of a possible self. The world that unfolds will be more vibrant and more profound.

Desire is central to this. Within the social worlds of gender that we fabricate, share, and commune with each other, we edge our bodies towards the unveiling of desire. Foregrounding generosity and reciprocity in communal contexts invites one to leave norms behind, to go deep with desires, flesh out fantasies, shift postures, and open oneself and one's worlds to change. The work of femmes teaches that committing to vibrancy (literally the vibration of the ensouled bodymind), care, and solidarity is necessary. We understand this as profoundly materialist – without the possibility to reject the expectations of gender(ed) normativity, or wage labour, one might not even tap into the sense of what they are drawn to, let alone how we may (re)assemble and grow together. Indeed, we recognise our complicity with these expectations and forms of work, as part of the process of forming an ethical life as part of the transformation through femme (social) life. Desire is not a single drive that propels us inevitably towards a pre-determined outcome. Desire is informed by sensuous and affective explorations, which vary in different contexts and relations. Desire is informed by safety and unsafety, by the possibility of making a getaway, or by inclusion into categories of desirability or relegation to ornamentation. Trans femmes face the desires of others which may come with undesirable curiosity.[7] Yet at other times, desire translates into expressions of openness and into play. Sometimes desire is the meat and two veg that helps us into the night, while in our dreams new vistas unfold for becoming in more leisurely times.

Meanwhile, neoliberalism aggressively demands that we become who we already are. We are made responsible for becoming likeable versions of ourselves that can offer niche productivity. Such productivity can be providing harmless diversity to colleagues, or emotional care for those who need it. It is said that we should do what we love, which often means that we must pretend to love what we do, in jobs that are not even likeable. When we do work that we like, we find that the conditions of that work systematically undermine our capacity to thrive. Between exploitation and these responsibilities, our affects and desires are caught in a tension between supporting us through the day, and being assaulted by marketing and other escapades of cruel optimism – directing us towards goals that will make us worse off.[8] The affective turn transformed wellness into an industry that demands we deal with ourselves as full agents in a world that is geared towards suppressing dissent. HR and PR departments blast us with a dreamscape of falsehoods, disembedded optimism, and marketable community. In these departments every formulation that we have collectively worked for is rehashed in glib statements that mock our intended meanings.

Yet we are who we are, and we don't become anything that we are not becoming together. Our emotions are attached to realities that need changing. In that sense, our affective and desiring life is profoundly material, and it is in this materiality that we find ways of relating that support navigating environments to influence our being in the world otherwise. We entangle with each other, and we engender each other.[9] In that mix of affirmation, resistance, and repulsion we make forms that hold our responsibility to each other carefully and with nuance. In this not knowing who *exactly* we are, what *exactly* we strive for, we find experiments of desire, affect, and meaning that are nevertheless grounded, material, and collective. By claiming we are who we are, we also claim a future that is entangled with our collective present selves, with a futurity that starts today, not in a promise of a better tomorrow. We change our lives not on the promise of a better life, but on the reality of how we live together. And we live with the question of how do you relate to us? Who am I for you? And we desire more open relations than we have experienced so far.

These questions profoundly invert the more masculine, at times policy-oriented question of 'how shall I relate to you?' That question wants answers about pronouns and pronunciations of names, while not addressing the empowerment of certain subjects. Collective agency is reduced to relatable answers from a single actor. The question is devoid of curiosity, invested instead in attempting to control a situation and leave oneself intact by harvesting some knowledge without vulnerability. Such is not our life. In femme life agency runs through the question of how one is treated, a question that is already collective. This disposition makes one approach the world responsively and responsibly.

As trans femmes who have been active in queer, trans and other political communities since the start of this century, we know that fixations on femininity are regularly met with debasement and disqualification, and at worst met with denigration and pathologisation. Institutional psychiatry and the Gender Clinic have historically only been interested in facilitating transition for trans women who display femininity that can be assimilated into a white, cis-normative, and heteronormative womanhood, which psychiatry conceives of as entailing sexual passivity; and for trans men who commit to masculinity and its expectations in work and life – for example to not become pregnant – where feeling better and being socially empowered are entangled. In addition, feminist movements and some queer movements invested in challenging patriarchal gender norms have displayed a tendency to read queer and trans femininities as socially regressive, condemning femmes and/or trans women. And white Western capitalist cultures have also been historically invested in visions of femininity as meekness, passivity, and oriented towards consumption, a gender expression opposed to a strong, virile, and empowered masculinity. While all three of these attitudes are outdated, their traces remain in our cultures and subcultures, and many people still read expressions of femininity as synonymous with weakness and conformity, see genders as oppositional, and confuse conformity with legitimacy.

However, over the last decade femme's consistent inventiveness transformed gender norms into a huge diversity of possibilities. Gendering practices by queer and trans femmes have never been so vibrant. (So vibrant that capitalism now wants a piece of it!) Together – plotting in the kitchen, assembling the grrrl gang and cycling through the streets – this means power is put to work towards the abolition of duress from gender norms, to transform and resist the violence enacted in the name of those norms. Within these communal contexts, femmes open up possibilities for how one connects with their body, dissolving the alienation of overdetermined binary expressions of gender, and the disconnections of isolating labour. Coming into the body emerges with the lifting of dysphoria (which is not merely the domain of pathologised transsexuals). Femme power emerges both at the level of one's body and in a communal/collective context, and these are interlinked.

FEMME IN THE COLLECTIVE

Through femme lives, through our friendships in the everyday, through the projects we forge, join and establish, we build collective power. At a social level, we check in on each other, on bodies and feelings, chemicals and processes, activities and relationships. We compare notes and experiences. We encourage self-expression in others, to experiment and try out looks, lives, desires. Through this, queer and trans and non-binary femmes forge and reaffirm bonds, friendships, relations, reaching out to hold differences and commonalities together. We create space to share, to eat together and cry with each other; to support and feel through the denigration and harm we (have) experience(d). We begin to scheme, to plot together, to organise on the smallest of levels (making art or food or clothes or zines) to the largest (building infrastructure and collectives). We lift each other up, celebrate big and small victories, such as achieving wins over institutions that have power over us or that have harmed us, of living in spite of racial capitalism. We hold up the joys of bodies, even if bodies are also sometimes hard to bear. We check in on healing; we build care teams to aid recoveries.

But femme life is not *just* about material transformation writ large in our local, personal, collective worlds. For us – the authors of this book – it's also about deepening the affects and the aesthetics of femininity and of gendering, understanding the interplay/influence of material conditions upon them. In the face of both economic *and* cultural austerity – the latter represented in austerity-chic and spartan purity and moralising[10] – femmes (femmes of colour in particular) pursue/embrace a sense of opulence, abundance and luxury, embellishing the worlds we've made together.[11] The turn outward to build joy, fun, desire, sensuality, together, comes with a turn inward to work through difficult emotions around our sense of self, our bodies, our desires, casting off shame or turning it into an aspect of sexual agency. Juana María Rodríguez waxes lyrical about her memories:

It was a magical sensory overload of music, movement, and the funk of flesh in heat. It was a huge, enveloping, color-filled closet, queer before queer was queer, fabulous and thrilling in my teenage eyes. And for about ten years, it was my everynight life, where I would go to dance and breathe in the possibility of queer life.[12]

This sensory overload is filled with possibility, its magic countering reasoned forms of becoming shaped by an entrepreneurial care
of the self as we might find in Aristotle or Foucault. Here is the
sensory envelopment of queer before queer was queer, queerness
is the future in the present, extending its arms in embrace. While
Rodríguez describes a process of learning dance by doing it collectively in Afro-Cuban migrant culture in the US, in her formulations
of non-discursive, non-analytic processes we recognise collective
processes of trans femme becoming. In contrast to the controlling
norms of feminisation, that may confront trans femmes, especially
in periods of transition, we recognise femme collective becoming in
the appreciation, encouragement, gestures, and support that nudge
us to embrace each other and brace for the world in unspoken scripts
of solidarity. We bear, broach, and hold space for the actions, knowledge, and perspectives of each other as survivors, coming to terms
with the harm that we've lived through and lived through our bodies.
We draw closer together in situations that are constricting, catch
each other's eyes in the crowd for support, and sense the sapping
of strength from our friend's bodies when they are under pressure.
We intuit each other's rhythms, perhaps to do with hormones, and
nudge reflection of the patterns that we sense. To share these experiences means that we have perspectives in common, and experiences
that tell us apart: each is part of the bond we share. We find means
to move through difficult affects (dysphoria, neglect, trauma, injury,
anger, etc.), identifying their sources in medical, familial, therapeutic, social, and institutional contexts – while situating these affects
in a wider context in which resources are restricted to a privileged
few, and sometimes needing professional support to work through
them. We learn from the femmes who have come before us, comparing *persistent* and *dangerous* desires, experiences, troubles and
passions. The emotional work we undertake opens up possibilities
in our bodies, and also in the social worlds we forge and share. We
crack open spaces to flourish, prepare the ground upon which to
sow flora and find company with fauna.

Domination in Europe functions through institutions and norms,
strutted up by anti-social hierarchies that impose epistemic and

social closure. (The role of institutions is discussed at length in Chapter 3.) To refuse these impositions, femme prioritises relationality as attentiveness, as care, as a way to openness. We work to oppose the abandonment and disposability of other marginalised people, as an abolitionist praxis, emerging in part from our own experiences of abandonment and disposability. In a political climate that is structured by intertwined xenophobia and institutional rights discourses, disposability is clearly visible on a national level through austerity and the response to the coronavirus pandemic, in which the basic operations of institutions are laid bare, shutting out some while enclosing others into their ranks.[13] We are hesitant to give up the sociality that we forged in nonnormative contexts, including the context of having had minimal rights. Entering institutions as full citizens demands compliance with structures that work against the solidarities that emerge in struggle. So we hesitate at the threshold of the institutions on which we are dependent for income, for work, for shelter. We learn to recognise the problems and patterns that occur in institutional contexts (including the family, the workplace, education, and medicine – not to be equated with care) and also in communities and in our social relations, problems that may reinforce the denigration of femmes, of our work or of our love.[14] But we also trace our own complicities.

Trans femme attentiveness aids the observation and analysis of our complicity in forms of life, because femme practices encourage action – to face frictions and work through problems in a way that opens up worlds to the rest of us. Speaking of complicity, Fred Moten writes:

I long for complicity. I don't want to stand out from the general complicity as if I were a bell, or a free and perfect moral agent, as if there were some space outside this shit where only special folks ungather one by one. That place in the sun was always *the* political fantasy, and now they say, to the folks to whom they refuse membership, that if you don't *want* to join, you ain't shit.[15]

The free and perfect moral agent is the individual around whom the institution is built. The idea of moral and epistemological perfection claims its own innocence and untouchability, and is detached from the context in which life is made; its lack of relation makes it prone to indifference, because it is fundamentally unsocial. Femmes sit with our complicit entanglements, facing the everyday mess that we navigate. The refusal of perfection leads to a refusal of innocence, and an embrace of sociality.

Femme entails the dissolution of structures that denigrate femininity. Femmeness makes a break with the problematic demands that shape normative (that is white, cis- and heteronormative, abled, and skinny) femininity, which include demands for certain forms of service, sexualisation, objectification, and also consumption. These demands and norms are made by agents of patriarchy, often husbands or fathers, bosses or managers, even the government. Women and LGBT people can also be guardians of the norm, often the price of inclusion – policing other women, queers, femmes and other feminised people, especially when it comes to race. Writing of the 'Rogue Femininity' of femme, Elizabeth Marston proposes 'that femme is dispossessed femininity'.[16] To be in the flow of the norms of gender may mean you exist to be available (to a husband or family), or that your femininity might be sold with your labour power (one might be good at a job because one learnt a skill that is expected by patriarchal norms of work discipline, or because one chooses to play to gender norms for cash). You may have to sell your labour power to reproduce the world as it is, cleaning it, feeding its children, caring for it, especially as a migrant, Black or Brown, feminised person.[17] To be dispossessed, in this case, is to be locked out of the capitalist relations that cohere in and through gender norms. You might be locked out of the family or the labour market, locked out of the gender binary or literally incarcerated by it,[18] locked out of your house or the place you were born, or all of these.

Femme is the stance when one didn't get domesticated by the norm, or maybe got broken by the norm, and emerges in consciously refusing alignment with it. In this split from the norm, femme femininities become unrecognisable and illegitimate, as they no longer draw on tropes of servitude and objectification. Femme femininities are not *for* the norm, but in defiance of it. It is the norm that, on the one hand, renders femmes invisible, unable to perceive what is considered perverse, and on the other hand affirms particular days of year for visibility (Lesbian Visibility Day, Trans Day of Visibility), where it is paying attention via algorithms. And, as Marston writes, in acts of passing one might choose to play the norm,[19] for whatever reasons we may have – be it for safety, for money, for a roof or for fun. At best, playing the norm is an act of strategic or tactical agency, and one in which we recognise our complicity with a norm that limits us. Defying the norm can take the highly pleasurable form of working through one's complicities, by giving up what may never have been not on the table in the first place. Towards making everyday lesbian, everyday trans.

The emotional work of care forms a sociality that subtends the public realm. Caring for other dispossessed people – other queer and trans folks, other marginalised people, the people that we build friendships and life with – shapes a more agential position. Care is about supporting each other's survival, towards flourishing. Thus, we don't want to give up care, because care is a mutual relation – what we give up is servitude.

FEMME SEXUALITY

In speaking of sexuality, we start at the top. What are the structural and social conditions affecting Black, Brown and white (trans) femme sexualities? Our communities and collectives exist under conditions of precarity, being overworked and under-employed, struggling with rent and crowdfunding healthcare. We repeatedly face social and institutional contexts where our self-expression, ideas, labour, and forms of being are dismissed, devalued, exploited, or abused. Nat has described this elsewhere as the conditions of transfeminine brokenness.[20] In addition, structural and historical forces of racism and white supremacy find their way into the social ecologies of queer and trans life. In both institutional and social contexts, transmisogynoir and whorephobia may run Black and

Brown trans femmes out of town – these are easier to pinpoint in social interactions, but more difficult to identify in the often more shielded domain of sexuality.

As we learn from Sharon Patricia Holland, writing about anti-Black racism in American social life and in queer theory's response to Black feminism, racism is at play all the way down.[21] Anti-Black racism feeds social anxieties regarding sexuality, manifesting on structural and interpersonal levels. It affects the very possibility of private life for Black and interracial relationships; it manifests intellectually when the writing of Black feminists on sexuality is left on the shelf to gather dust, or not integrated into analysis of feminist sexual practices that emerged during the sex wars. Holland argues that the autonomous desiring subject posited in queer theory is implicitly encoded as white, male, and we would add cis and able-bodied; and that the conditions of desiring for Black queer females are imbricated in familial forms where (heteronormative) social and sexual reproduction can't as easily be laid by the wayside. The same could be used to describe South Asian family forms, although there is also a marginal history in which queer women couples might fit into these forms, particularly in lower and middle castes.[22] This is not to say that Black and Brown families and communities are more socially conservative than white ones (that old trick) – it is instead to say that the imaginary that progress for LGBTQ people comes through reforming conservative social forms by recognition of legal rights encodes whiteness in a manner that may not transfer to ethnic or diasporic communities, and which in turn affects the expectations placed upon Black, Brown and other minority ethnic queer and trans femmes.

Juana María Rodríguez teaches us to think about the material conditions undergirding sexual relations of Latina femmes and other femmes of colour. Rodríguez describes how women of colour have faced sexual sacrifice through shame and censure, encouraged to forego pleasure for 'communal respectability' and 'the common good'.[23] She points to how non-reproductive sexual activities have faced pathologisation and criminalisation, while women of colour and disabled people have also been subjected to eugenic practices and sterilisation.[24] Negotiating the tensions of sexuality and social respectability, amidst state policing and control of bodies, is a challenge of inventing practices, especially in a context of limited representations of what is possible. This is supported by generously sharing knowledge and speaking into silence, with the need to steadfastly develop verbal and non-verbal means of communication. Rodríguez speaks vividly of the roles of gesture, dance and fantasy in service of this.

The desires of trans and other femmes may be sidelined within our social ecologies – in terms of who we desire sexually, what kinds of ensouled bodyminds and what kinds of lives. Even radical social ecologies, or those rooted in collectivity, can tend towards the reproduction of normative forms – be that through queer and trans social reproduction and care, who gets checked-in on and who gets checked out. When we reground social ecologies by changing how and where we meet, eat, and move together and how we relate to and understand the ground on which we stand, we are working with the *play* of social forms. This might occur through creative spaces or events, for instance, a performance or a screening that questions the objectification of trans femmes or places front and centre our sexual agency. It may be a conversation that is steered by the need to talk about consent, or the discomfort when sex-positive spaces reproduce forms of exclusion through the valorisation of abled, skinny, white, or queer masculinities, over and above other bodies or forms of expression. In the spirit of challenging expectations, working to undo the racial and gendered, cissexist, ableist, fatphobic, xenophobic, ageist economies can open space for expression, although we might find these social pressures wired more deeply within us than we expected.

Sexuality is a key element of coming to know one's body, from learning and understanding sensations, pleasures, and difficulties, to undoing the norms and expectations of social conservativism and shame. This is part of the reason why conservative and neoliberal political programmes work ideologically to suppress and control knowledge and expressions of sexuality (often under the guise of protecting vulnerable people and minors). The neoliberal era

22

of LGBTQ Rights has also worked to keep sexual expression and deviance in the home and behind closed doors, unless it involves sex work (where we see pushes towards criminalising sex workers or clients, and making working conditions more risky for sex workers) or the sexual expression of Black, Brown and Indigenous people (who still get policed, harmed, and sometimes killed in the privacy of their/our homes).[25] When it comes to discourses around transness, the push for respectability and assimilation has left sexuality out of the equation. This may in part be due to appeals going back to the 1990s to separate public conceptions of transsexuality from 'sexuality' – to locate transness in the space of gender – although queer transfeminists of that period also pinned their kinks to their chests.[26] Moreover, this was in the context of the active pathologisation of trans desires and sexuality by psychiatry since the mid-twentieth century. However, by the early 2010s, trans folks still faced an inquisitive, violent curiosity regarding genitals – trans activists (liberals and radicals) undergirded this was no one else's business; although trans liberalism promised that if society would include us, like 'everyone else', we'd also behave respectably (especially when invited into the Houses of Parliament). Shifting the conversation to rights (trans people's marital rights and legal gender recognition) overshadowed everyday conversations about sexuality, about abortion, and, initially, about getting pregnant. Like queer liberalism before it, the sanitised reframing of trans and non-binary folks might make some of us more respectable, but often at the expense of those of us who wear our sexualities upon our sleeves, or those of us who are objectified and hyper-sexualised (most often Black and Brown trans women and other trans people of colour). We are well aware that sanitised contemporary trans representation, the hypersexualisation and objectification of trans women within pornography aimed at men,[27] and the lack of discourse around trans sexuality outside of queer and trans zine culture have real material effects upon us.[28] Cultural imaginaries do affect how desirable and datable other people find us, and this in turn affects our positions within economies of care.

Openness about sexuality allows for a social awareness of who might want/need/desire something out of need, necessity, or sense of safety. To be 'someone's first trans femme lover' is at times harrowing and navigating 'the big reveal' of genitals can be anxiety-provoking. How to invent a way to navigate the (im)possibility of relating to trans genitals – which are by social pressure mimetically gesturing to cis-binaries, rather than existing as simply a bodily part? Sex is not about *what* is in your underwear; it's about sensation, play, being cognisant of pleasure, but also discomfort and hang-ups too. Intersex and trans people are more interested in emphasising the diversity of genitals, rather than obsessing over and fetishising them or classifying them according to a binary. The sexual short courses on how to be touched and how not, and gently explaining where to lube, when to undress, consent, and all of this tactfully while not breaking the sexual atmosphere, can be disheartening or depressing, or fun and exhilarating – whether it is, is often a matter of skill and trust.

T4t relationality – that is trans people desiring, dating, and having sex with other trans people – can contribute to undoing the norms which mark certain trans bodies as undesirable, unspooling desire from cis-normative standards of beauty and attractiveness, proposing different sexual practices, and potentially different life goals and vectors of futurity. Grounded in the sweetness of a commonality of trans experience or of trans and queer subcultures, t4t begins with genders or bodies otherwise, without such experiences being identical, even if at times there are similarities. Beauty and desire look and feel different, sometimes ditching the 'classical' standards of feminine or masculinity completely; relationships become a space of opportunities for expression and play, where assuredness, presence, and pleasure may have previously been denied or neglected. T4t relationality affirms that trans lives entail explorations and shifts in one's life direction, or temporal disruptions, when compared with normative, bourgeois life trajectories of growth, age and change – as sexual and gender orientations and bodies can change, and such change requires time and energy.

Social dynamics do not overdetermine sexual dynamics. While in queer relationships, an interplay of femme and butch dynamics is not overdetermined by gender expression, t4t can emphasise the creative character of sexual dynamics even more. When it comes to sex, queer erotics involving the whole body connect to a multiplicity of orifices, appendages, prosthetics, and genitals too. Touch becomes a practice (or a method) of exploring what is exciting or pleasurable. Consent remains important; and sometimes pain becomes part of the mix too – potentially functioning to acknowledge and hold space for what has been lived through. Language and gesture, both verbal and non-verbal, can become means of (re)coding and (re)inscribing bodies according to what is felt and desired. Indeed, we have lived and known a multiplicity of bodies – in spite of preconceived ideas of what trans bodies are, or how they 'should' be according to pathology or institutional gender standards. There is no singular trans femme embodiment, as with other trans and non-binary embodiments.

Femmeness encourages us to approach sex as agents of our own pleasure and care; while also recognising that coming into one's sexuality isn't easy. Sex requires vulnerability as well as experimentation. We learn the centrality of negotiating consent with partners and in play; to make safer conditions of risk and care. We recognise the reparative power in sexual practices – to challenge abjection, shame, dysphoria, and dissonance – where we are able to negotiate and work with presence and (dis)comfort with our bodies, and to explore the trajectories through which we as ensouled bodies have travelled. Body change, and the (re)presentation of one's body, may lead to setting off fireworks – the experience of struggle consummated in pleasure. But this depends on one feeling cared for and heard by sexual partners, not always a given or something that comes easily. Sex requires check-ins. Our trauma interrupts us in unexpected ways. A guiding touch can bring us back. We get lost and find our way to return. Simultaneously we hold our partners and navigate their history and interruptions, transforming the norms that were enforced upon our bodies to make play a healing escape, a revisitation, and a mode of comforting each other.

With an emphasis on openness – to deep knowledge, to living and being otherwise, to connect into reciprocal relations of care – femme holds open space to tune into, share and shift towards one's desires. We propose that the emotional space for desiring is one that depends upon care – upon having one's *needs* met – in the first instance. If communities or individuals are focused on day-to-day survival, the idea of dreaming big, of holding space for fantasy and imagination, may never make it onto the agenda. Indeed, this is a dynamic we have witnessed ourselves – fighting state racism and supporting our disabled, trans and queer friends amid the violence of austerity politics and the coronavirus pandemic will always trump opportunities to dream. Our ensouled bodyminds end up in crisis mode, coping with the pains of trauma, trying to make ends meet and pay the rent. We're left to work ourselves to the bone, trying to rest enough, with maybe finding a moment to feed on culture. To go deep into an analysis or expression of sexuality demands time to tap into oneself or to seduce a lover. Finding space for depth may entail making time in the bedroom, or creating a public space; going beyond needs into the pursuit of pleasure. Where pleasure is not subjugated to the demands of activism against the structures that attempt to overpower us, pleasure can be a source of energy and bonding for this activism.

COMPLICITY AND FRICTION, IN AND BETWEEN COLLECTIVES

Across this book, we discuss how (trans) femmeness approaches collectivity and its attendant problems. We focus on collectivity in juxtaposition to the term community. Community is used in many different ways, but we understand it to mean a social group where there is something that group members have in common, but one doesn't necessarily know everyone. Collectives, on the contrary, exist through direct relations between people. It is a term that emerges for us from left-wing organising or the squat movement. Collectives are often horizontally organised; and working with frictions in collectives is a key part of learning to organise. This includes dealing with finding oneself the problem, without lapsing into guilt, defending ignorance, or hoping for a world in which innocence is an option.

We think about complicity, because we live in worlds in which we are interlinked in many ways – not all of them voluntary, consensual or desired. We enter into worlds that are imposed on us, such as the economically Hostile Environment that forces us into jobs we might not want.[29] In this world, we may need to display professional behaviour that we do not consent to (for instance, to greet all customers, with courtesy and a smile, while one is mistreated by their boss, or to participate in the professionalisation of trans studies); or be instructed to align with institutional demands that we cannot always stop (we might resist Prevent screenings,[30] or mandatory attendance monitoring for visas, but teachers still need to grade their students even if from a pedagogical perspective we find the practice irrelevant or even harmful). In doing the work of uprooting structures that enclose us in harmful ways, we need to attend to the way these structures find form within us and in our collectives. We do not undertake this work from a critical distance, but primarily through making different forms of life. Debarati Sanyal understands complicity as a 'structure of engagement that produces ethical and political reflection across proliferating frames of reference'.[31] We take engagement to mean the practice of making new forms of living, to make sure we are not forced into a single way of knowing the world. In these forms of living otherwise, we find pleasure and joy where we meet, love, have sex, organise, and make sense of what matters.

These different worlds – the hegemonic and those we fabricate with each other – are not cleanly separated, nor are the worlds we make for ourselves free from friction. While Kai Cheng Thom comments playfully and self-critically on 'the revolutionary over-enthusiasm of university queers', who want to go off with painted hair and raise unicorns on a collective farm,[32] we don't question dreams of living apart from the contemporary world. The worlds we live in are made with shared references, different viewpoints, experiences, and also contain everyday frictions between each other, as well as dealing with normative duress. In the worlds we create collectively, we might find ourselves in situations where we are part of a problem or are a problem for someone else; sometimes, we are the problem for ourselves. And while resisting imposed worlds, we may find ourselves walked over by the bravado of comrades; or we might escape into a collective in which we enjoy ourselves, but that remains unreachable to others. It might be that our individual pleasures disrupt a collective. We often cannot solve the problems that are created by structures, and we might bring problems back home. The issue of complicity presents itself in both institutional settings, and in situations where we act collectively. We need to think through complicity to deal with the many points of reference that we bring to the table, that we meet in our lives, and as reminder to face what needs to be faced rather than ignore it.

Some collectives strive for purity by searching for the 'right rules' or 'proper' deference against (at times generalised) experiences of oppression, as a way to cope with social complexities. The move towards decontextualised narratives happens because we cannot always share our personal experiences with groups, or we cannot do so without collapsing into gestures of representation, where sometimes our individual experiences represent the experiences of those deemed to fit our category. But new norms of what constitutes a proper response to duress can be alienating. Because I'm trans my experiences are perhaps about trans, until it appears they don't fit the current style and rules of discussion. Experience-led organising can collapse into an obligation to testify, and this testimony must be delivered in a recognisable and prescribed format.

A becoming that aims to escape from imposed categories might ask for a 'divestment of codes and signification, of identity, and taking on the register of the impersonal'.[33] This divestment needs an air of depersonalisation, while in contrast we as femmes seek to embellish and shine. But more (de)pressingly, such divestment asks us to relay our experiences as if they are unique, which sadly they are not. Social pressure is often impersonal. Furthermore, the collectivity that we crave against isolation and disposability relies on mutual recognition as well as the possibility of differentiation. So, we revert to structural analysis, avoiding the soul-destroying imperative to demonstrate our pain as an individualisation of identity.

The technique of critique, as an examination of the limits we run up against, is the primary method by which we make a case for a better life.[34] But if or when one attains a better life, and one's politics are not informed by direct pain – what then? We see, for instance, such a pattern with education. When one is not formally educated, as is the case for one of our grandparents, access to education is a matter of struggle. But when the descendants of those deprived of formal education are able to access it, the familial memories of struggle are called into question and one's own experience is easily dismissed as 'privilege'. Such approaches narrowly focus on direct experiences of oppression, rather than a multiplicity of experiences, frames of reference and generational memories. Multiplicities of experience muddle such categorical homogeneity and disrupt a politics of purity.[35] Assuming identities are homogenous allows for clear policies and rules that require no relational approaches. Decontextualising allows rules that create the appearance of a grip on reality. Rules soon become the reality, and contexts and collectives disappear under rules, norms, and policies, satisfying a craving for stability. Even well-intended guidelines can substitute imagined realities for lived experiences, and in the process homogenise groups and give those who adhere to rules a false sense of, what we would call exaggeratedly, innocence. Innocence suggests one is not creating limits for others, nor limiting oneself.[36] Social or institutional regulations can provide a false sense of security because they exist at a remove from the socialities that make reality sticky, and murky and thereby needing attentiveness. Rules in this sense allow for organisational speed and crowd control.[37] They also individualise action, because if you stick to the rules, you are not guilty. Institutional policies claim to protect staff that follow their protocols, regardless of the violence they may dispense, which is especially clear in policing, armies, and internment but also medical ethics.[38] However, the structure of rules is not only present inside institutions, but also outside of them. We see it in everyday interactions that are undoubtedly streamlined by, say, the regulatory ethos encouraged by social media.

Debarati Sanyal explains complicity as being folded into a situation – not standing on the sidelines (perhaps looking at the guilty one who transgressed the rules, perhaps shaming them), but rather a call to action and shared responsibility for a situation (and how it might be changed).[39] This combines with the attentiveness at the heart of our transfeminism – highlighting forms of care that not only attend to needs, reproduction, or survival, but also to a reality to ensure it is not curbed by discursive categories.[40] Such attentiveness is saturated with the possibilities of exchange that occur in close proximity. Thinking about complicity helps us, on the one hand, to see positionality as a marker that determines the demands of hegemonic structures on our lives, and on the other hand, indicates how our becoming and our politics shape our understandings, relations, relatability, and attention. Structural politics makes demands on how we share experiences, shed light on situations, and 'speak from our position' – and sometimes this demands stasis, rather than allowing our insight to develop with others in diffuse and intermingled collectives. We work through how we appear and how others relate to us, and how power plays into this, including our own power and how we use it. Because some parts of our lives are not accessible to all. And when we meet people who have been shut out by the norm, we might find that we cannot hold space for everyone in each collective, or we find that our form of living is alienating to some. It might show how norms pop up inside of collectives, that shut some people out; and that the bonds that help us make it through, are experienced by some as obstacles, intentionally or unintentionally. Or that the political struggles of our parents enable different lives for us or access to institutions, while this access can make us forget the solidarities and cultures forged through their struggles.[41] Thinking through complicity reminds us of the struggles of past generations, to counter the normalisation (and depoliticisation) we have arrived at.

We also claim we are part of the problem because other people make us the problem. We bring social problems into situations, where people scrutinise us, judge us, or feel the need to be 'very open' to us in ways that are not always comfortable. It makes no sense to claim the problem is merely 'elsewhere' and we are 'innocent' of it. We might not be innocent – we might have pre-figured responses to instances of what, for instance, appears to be transmisogyny, that go beyond what a situation requires. We might have stores of anger ready to share, or feel defeated before we really are, we might in words hear echoes that others do not. We are not exculpated of any given problem, our culpability is something that needs to be navigated.[42]

However, there is a clear difference between people who are closed out by nonnormative collectives, for instance by racism, and people who (perhaps inadvertently) close themselves off to certain perspectives, experiences of duress, or modes of solidarity. The claim to complicity functions very differently on each side of the break – complicity in practices that push people out invites a different manner of reflection than complicity with those same practices when one is themself closed out. Evoking Thom, this does not mean that we side with a liberal vision, which claims that truth lies in the middle.[43] Rather, in social justice work we are collectively responsible for the way we interact, even if it means that we cannot always solve the problems emerging directly in specific interactions. It means honouring the enormous amount of labour it takes to create trust in collectives. The hurt of being closed out of a place where one hoped to flourish and find companionship is real, after all.

Neoliberalism disrupts trust in collectives, and a lack of relational skills can lead to breakdowns in communities. The sensuous is one space where friction can be circumvented (we expand on this below). Friction indicates points where worlds do not overlap. Some members of a group may be aware that their needs are deviating from this particular collective – sometimes because of their overlaps with other groups, or since they come with different histories and needs.[44]

There is no withdrawing into a form of life which allows us to avoid structural problems. The problems of trans life – from the interwoven pressures of racism, xenophobia, ableism, and misogyny to mutual frictions caused by structural stress and precarity – inhibit simple ways of coping. This defies the frictionless policy-based hopes of liberalism. To embrace complicity is to interrupt the space-making practices imposed by normative binary gendering. Binary norms pair transgression and agency with victimisation and passivity. Due to the passive nature of the 'victim', or so the story goes, an external force is required to intervene and protect the innocent harmed one. Innocence introduces force, and force demands allegiance with power: this is why the performance of innocence is necessary. It is the renewal of the bond with institutionalised force. The entire model of individualisation retains the structure that requires the existence of perpetrators, police, and judgements. Centring complicity as sociality, as conspiracy,[45] dashes the liberal hope for a frictionless space of innocence. For liberals, such a space promotes adherence to a single order and creates the policing function of management: hierarchy and control are required elements, introducing coercion for some, and a smooth ride for those in charge. Stepping into the fray of social life requires embracing that we act, because actions make patterns, and that these patterns might need to be changed to create openness to difference, rather than separability. To face that is to ask how we can show up for each other and how do we make and facilitate spaces.

TENSIONS THREADING FABRICS OF WORLDS – COMPLICITY AND SOLIDARITY

The sensuous entangles multiple worlds, by highlighting that our needs are not homogenous group requirements; sensing underlines we need different relations and forms of sociality that support our survival and connection. Embracing the sensuous complexity of worlds as a form of understanding complicity also shapes how we understand solidarity. Solidarity manifests through making forms that work towards collective and total liberation, as we discuss in Chapter 5. Furthermore, liberation does not lead to a friction-free existence. In a world that is multiple, collisions form the building blocks of new forms.

There are two sides to our thinking about complicity. First is finding the right relation to your position in the world. In white responses to structures of duress, one's relation to one's position in the world is often interrelated with guilt, but finding the right relation is more interesting than that. It entails attending to where one is, and what one can do from that place. From that contextualisation, one can determine when one is responsible for stepping in, for creating/supporting collective resistance, or contributing ideas to the collective domain. The right relation is not quite the same as positionality. Where positionality refers to a structural situatedness, the right relation is directional, applying agency from where one is. Femme relational approaches avoid conflating the various layers of life with a general structure, in part by being attentive to socialities. Conflation of the social with generalisations leads to immobilisation, rather than activation of one's agency. For a theory of oppression, a totalising account might be impressive. However, it does not lead to a focus on resistance, as María Lugones reminds us.[46]

Finding the right relation entails questioning roles and practices in a communal context. Focusing on practices connects embodied action with (liberating) imaginaries, rather than hiding actions under structuring rules, claiming that the rule is the problem and denying translation of rules into actions. An embodied approach that links action, knowledge and forms has been termed a somatechnical approach.[47] Somatechnics means a reliance on ways of relating that are held communally and bodily. In this context that means placing one's being amidst modes of relating that support the collective. While rules rely on generalising terms that traverse different contexts, relations are in flux and differences are always situational. Relationality is contextual, whereby differences not only remain intact but can even flourish. Attention to context, including structural and generalising pressures, enables thinking about complicity by delineating relations that might not be emancipatory. Sometimes, this discussion takes shape as a focus on privilege, but it is wider – it comes with dominating imaginaries, disconnecting sensoria, local empowerment and misreading of actions.

The second, more positive side of thinking through complicity centres openness to alliances, friction and arguments, a readiness to question the organisation of practices. This openness to tensions informs a view of the structure of relations. In rule-guided organisations, tension signifies a breakdown. In collectives, to embrace tension, the possibility emerges of enhancing openness. Embracing complicity without guilt gives room for experiment, play, embellishment, and new senses of joy. A willingness to change without guilt or defensiveness can dissolve the hostilities that are sometimes present across fault lines. Friction in collectives highlights not necessarily tensions between hegemony or normativity and nonnormativity, but the points where collectives close themselves off from making connections. Sometimes, such friction can be extra hurtful, for instance, because the collective was a 'first home', or made new things possible, or was a space of safety that feels shattered. Being open to acknowledging such complicities is a starting point for addressing difficult tensions – they are not solved simply by an analysis of social hierarchy (even if that can play a role). Working with and through tensions, as in instances of queer, trans and/or femme world-making, is less a set of critical actions that clear up misunderstandings in the existing order, such as rule-based accounts purport to do, as it is a sensuous opening to ways of worlding.

Thinking and living trans femme sociality entails embracing new forms of life that are not absorbed into the norm. However, some of our practices (including nonnormative ones) still may create problems, practices that sometimes nevertheless feel good to us. Such practices may need to be retuned and not thrown out completely. Relationality is about practice in many senses of the word, including how practices become embodied and how that embodiment may obscure its own closedness and reproduction of duress (for instance, in dominant bodies coming together to constitute social groups). This can create the conditions of embodied disconnection or separation, by reifying emotional and sensorial differences, epistemic differences, experiential differences, or different histories.[48] Sometimes, the disconnect in marginalised bodies occurs from being out of sync with, or overwhelmed by, one's context or surroundings. In complex collectives, these differences cannot necessarily be 'solved'. Simultaneously, such disconnect may indicate where we need to hold on – to invoke Denise Ferreira da Silva – to be different without reproducing separability.[49] Holding differences can be exhilarating and inspiring, can enhance understanding and complexity, and can keep open spaces when homogeneity would close them.

CARE IN THE COLLECTIVE WORLDS –
RECEIVING LABOUR, OFFERING GENEROSITY

Yet, to focus on agency alone in remaking ways of worlding misses that there are also other tensions at stake. A lot of people want to give, but don't want to receive. Leah Lakshmi Piepzna-Samarasinha draws attention to this problem.[50] People join collectives – for instance, mutual aid groups early in Spring 2020 during the coronavirus pandemic – because they are ready to be supportive, but while joining they rely either on a private structure of care or will never ask for help. This lack of mutuality can reaffirm the racial and gendered divisions of labour under capitalism that structures care – where marginalised Black, Indigenous, brown, feminised, disabled, trans, queer and/or migrant people bear the burden of much of the world's care work in waged and institutional relations, and in social relations.[51] Those who are less marginalised amid these relations will also need less care. Self-sufficiency is an enduring mythical aspiration[52] of racial capitalism – which itself depends on material relations that are interrelated across the globe, relations that reproduce unequal divisions of labour, the exploitation of people, labour, land, 'natural resources' and more, all of which are rooted in colonial dispossession.[53] The drive to support others from a position of self-sufficiency, while either refusing or seemingly not needing to receive care, reproduces a dynamic of philanthropy – 'I am "generous" with the wealth/capital/labour/skills I have accumulated (or hoarded) and will do good or fund activities to reproduce the world as I see it (from my colonial bourgeois imperialist position)'.[54] Affluent white people (those who have resources) in organisations or collectives run to 'solve' problems (that is, throw money/time at these problems while not addressing their structural causes), reproducing this dynamic of white supremacy. Meanwhile, marginalised folks find ourselves dislocated in a world of the privileged, while fighting and struggling to maintain our own worlds, our bodyminds, our lives. So how can interdependence arise when worlds of care are interrupted or under duress? At the same time, we see that an insistence on structural privilege fixes the roles of giver or taker of care, while pressures or contingencies of life uproot fixed positions.[55]

Working in large groups with a communal structure is not for everybody. A lot of time is spent talking to create space for decision-making; to make such spaces work as a whole, there's a lot of unacknowledged femme labour in the background. The collective is made in the 'little work' of femme labour. As Piepzna-Samarasinha writes, 'Our organizing skills [...] are incredible, and often not respected as much as masculine leaders', or indeed seen as skills'.[56] When the labour of organising sociality disappears, communal structures tend not to hold up, letting go of the bodies they support.[57] Confidence in decision-making is not how everybody works, and definitely not how groups work. Giving can be about giving attention, rather than sharing insights, and receiving is equally about receiving words as it is about finding an attentive ear.

If femme labour or care is not present or has been driven out, organisations become a different kind of structure: they may cohere into a centralised structure, or decisions become forms of power play. Sometimes it is better if a group disbands itself and ceases to be. Sociality helps to band together *and* to disband collectives. A femme sociality can support unlearning hegemony, by opening us to other forms that surround us. Unlearning can be a preparation against the pushy demands of hegemony, of whiteness, of patriarchy. Or unlearning can entail not knowing what to do yet, encouraging us to mix what we know to do with what we haven't experienced (yet) – requiring sharing knowledge and reflecting on its limits. María Lugones explains hegemony as a world where 'his sense is the only sense'.[58] Moving away from this logic of purity – that is a logic of control – we step into a sense of being able to let go of what we bring, stalling it, to pick it up later perhaps. We are looking to allow the gaps in our experience to support mutuality, with the right kind of openness to what we don't know (rather than the 'right kind of knowledge'). Learning what we don't know requires engaged listening and reflecting on what might be overlooked in a collective. Embracing such attentiveness is an act of resistance, as Lugones has laid out, when she names it a 'social commentary'.[59] Such commentary is only possible in the context of a sociality that is open to different senses.

Femme practices do not lean on a single order of being in the world: they are not singly logical, sensorial, or affective. Different connections are made and grow into new practices. The refusal to reduce worlding to a single sense (e.g. the visual or the logical) allows worlding to become 'luxurious'. This luxuriousness, opulence, or abundance is an openness to meaning and connection. Conversely, singular, normative approaches frame themselves with scarcity, as purifying practices restrict the cross-pollination of worlds, creating competition between explanations, understanding and points of view. When one's world consists of a single logic, one is asked to give up all one has; but in a world saturated with an abundance of connections, such generosity is merely a way to renew one's sense of connection. It (almost) doesn't matter what logic I bring – in the moment I start to *impose* it, I become the problem. The moment one is ready to dissolve a single order, complicity becomes complexity.

RETURNING INTUITIONS AND REWIRING THE SENSUOUS

Neoliberalism is a politics of indifference[60] that strengthens authoritarian structures, reinforcing commodified institutional logics. In this 'Hostile Environment' (xenophobic politics are always a mirror of how states treat citizens), care can function as an attentiveness to differences and different ways of worlding. In a sensuous materialism (informed by José Esteban Muñoz), Joshua Chambers-Letson writes, 'commensurability, necessary for market exchange, flattens the sensuous and detailed nature of life as it is actually lived'.[61] Writing about the sensuous awareness of world-making in its serious and playful forms, Chambers-Letson reminds us that knowledge concerns both risk and play, and is not limited to the articulable. Knowledge is also practical, and skilful, rather than exclusively verbal, where risk and play in practice, thinking, and action influence how one navigates social spaces. Femme embellishment taps into playful and serious sensual awareness, encouraging shifts in one's focus and staying open to the world.

Gloria Anzaldúa indicates that it is usually the ego which commands the focus of the senses.[62] This commanding focus gets generalised into 'common sense', leading to actions that reproduce dominant structures. Responsibility requires the difficult acknowledgement that one's intuition about how to do things may at times be wrong. Rewiring the sensory entails a retuning of the intuitive. This rewiring is (in part) conscious, involving presence and gentleness – and it undoes the essentialist idea that intuition is a singular thing. Furthermore, intuition is an important part of not being alienated from oneself. One does not 'have' an intuition – intuition emerges from one's connection to environments, and how one interplays with the world.[63]

When we sense that something is wrong, our sensing is by no means indifferent to duress and at times aligns with it. Sometimes this alignment is direct, bringing institutional practices or the institution itself into spaces where people have tried to keep it out or to work against it. In a drive that emerges as hunger[64] – in spaces where relationality is stripped away – intuition works to pull a person through. This can be a hunger to be alive, a hunger for a different life, for a different sociality that opens up another sense of the world – this is what transness is, lived in and through the body and the world(s). Transness is not rebellion against what is preordained by god or nature (as if we are restaging the Enlightenment). Transness is a different hunger, as A. Sivanandan would perhaps agree, a hunger for a life not lived yet, that we are rehearsing in the underground.[65] Stuart Hall reminds us that this strategy is 'Another [face] – principled, militant, intransigent in opposition: yet gentle in personal relationship – is reserved for comrades and friends with whom [one] has become linked and bound in struggle, "below ground"'.[66] We are with each other, we do not abandon each other to the demands of the institution, but intuitively feel our way out.

The retuning of intuition may be conceived as one aspect of a rewiring of the sensuous that femmeness inaugurates. Through institutional critique and decoloniality; embracing the lines of attention and flight that come with queer and trans femme desires – from one's gaydar, to the desire to be strapped up and fucked or to fuck in certain ways; to finding new ways to hold friendships; to the drive to abolish patriarchal and racist conservative institutions such as the nuclear family or Gender Clinic; through the worlds and ways of life we forge and hold together; to the ways we collectivise our care labour for the remaking of our ensouled bodyminds and somatechnics, refusing the disposability of marginalised bodies; to the politicised aesthetics and joy we derive from our deep recognition and embrace of rogue, abject, and/or high femininity. We come to know the politics in our queer desires that draw out attention otherwise.[67] We mobilise all of these to dethrone racial capitalism in our everyday lives, on the streets, and even in our labour relations. As we learn from Sean Bonney and Kirsten Ross, during the height of the 1871 Paris Commune, Rimbaud proposed the necessity for poets to 'cultivate' the soul through 'a long, immense and logical derangement of all the senses. All forms of love, suffering, and madness'.[68] Rimbaud endeavoured in that historical moment to undo the grip of empire on the soul through the senses. In this spirit, we propose that anti-colonial femmes are in the work of rewiring our senses anew – in and through our ensouled bodyminds (unlearning Cartesian separations), situated and in relation to the worlds we make together and that we need and desire.[69] This rewiring can be supported by hormones, as Eva Hayward, speaking of taking Premarin, describes how one's *proprioceptive sense is as radically changed* as external presentation'.[70] While a change of soma under medicalised and Cartesian frames is conceived as the only cure for the transsexual mind, Hayward underlines how the 'expressive potential of the body, its capacity to respond to the world, is substantively modified, transforming the sensuous exchange of self and environment'.[71] Undoing and unfeeling an assigned body and normative manners of embodiment (which were perhaps never intuitive), comes through body-conscious and chemical transformation. Although, this has implications for one's material relations and exchange with one's surroundings. You still need to find a presence in a world, where one is held through relation. Femme is a mode of relational solidarity, questioning the Enlightenment desire to possess.[72] Decolonization undermines the material relations of capitalism that we were taught.[73]

Femme ethics is not about what to claim, but how to relate and how to be/make that are stake. We desire luxuriousness and abundance, good food, ever-opening relationality and world-travelling (by way of Lugones) – in the face of organised scarcity and dispossession under racial capitalism, which only understands abundance as the hoarding of material wealth. We modify the demand from the 2018 Women's Strike – 'Bread and Roses for All, and Hormones Too'[74] – planting new shoots for food and flowers, even if our gardens are grown on top of concrete, or amid high-rise buildings. We grow into lives we were warded off from; we make gardens with the friends we were once taught to avoid. We desire and love each other, other queers and other trans people, in the face or our denigration and abjection from norms and institutions. We love amid the refusal of their logics of value (and social capital). Hard is this love and we love hard.

Participants in nonnormative forms of life become skilled in existing across different worlds simultaneously. Lugones termed this 'world-travelling', an idea that rests on the building and moving between different worlds. Femmeness creates spaces where sensing can be opened up to the different layers between worlds, where sensing itself can be multitudinous. Trans femme worlding is a collective practice that reaches out beyond the mire of the present, the 'prison house' of the 'here and now',[75] proposing the future is now. Why wait for inclusion in a neoliberal form – that, as we discuss in Chapter 3, promises little in rights and security, and doesn't seem to want to really include us – when it is possible and *necessary* to shape forms of living in the present that reflect life in a way we want to live it. Here, in practice, we try forms of life that enhance solidarity and that bring some worlds closer. Sometimes practices, or collectives, fail, and we learn from their mistakes. The emphasis on practice means that it is not a way of knowing that is at stake, but a way of making worlds that in turn supports changes in ensouled bodyminds, where reflection follows action; we learn by moving across worlds with care and attentiveness to different positions and hirstories.

The practices of embracing complicity and complexity as generous, attentive care, link to the abolition of structures of duress in their punitive form. Carceral technologies function to keep a single order in place, through their suppression of rebellion and redistribution, and expansion of racial criminalisation. We see hegemony as the impetus to dominate through practices that disconnect; we understand social justice work as relating to undoing structures of separation – which does not mean we have to form a single collective into which everybody fits. Ensuring we do not base our practices of responding to each other in hierarchy, unity, functionality, or policing requires rethinking how forms of life are maintained. Generously opening forms and embracing different manners of sense-making, is a reprieve from the exhausting demands and divisions of labour and life, of land and bodies, under capital. Within femme worlds, solidarity holds out the possibility of rewiring of one's senses, retuning our intuitions into the frequencies of our complicities; different flowers come into bloom.

2

Transfeminist ethics and practices of care

LANDING IN TRANS LIVES AS THEY ARE LIVED

Under the pressures of needs and necessity, we make, maintain, and fight for our lives – responding, organising, and living with resistance. We share the skills necessary for collective living, self-building homes off-grid, joining housing co-operatives, making lives possible through care collectives, sharing material resources to secure housing, squatting, unionising workplaces, being jobless, being on welfare, drawing on various languages, figuring out how things work in new countries, living in a collective or large shared house due to high rents, community education, being homeless, having nothing to fall back on except community resources for mental healthcare or food or personal assistance, learning how institutions work, or making a toxic urban environment liveable. It is the challenges of material conditions that leave poor and precarious, disabled and abled, racialised and/or migrant and/or white queer and trans people with different and intensive care needs. We find ourselves more vulnerable to harm and in need of other ways of living.[1] This chapter addresses collective care as a practice of interdependent survival and the forging of meaningful relations as a means towards liberation, while elaborating an ethics that emphasises solidarity and support, attentiveness and love. We understand that transfeminist care and ethics hold collective practices together that elaborate alternative worlds and ways of living. This ethics entails the refusal of disposability and devaluation of marginalised people that is encouraged within neoliberal capitalism, by focusing on how we are navigating and transforming the space left open by institutional neglect.

Considering the differences between care in collectives and institutional contexts reveals the conditions under which the necessity for collective care is continually (re)produced, as an antidote to the dynamics of institutional care. We focus on collective and community dynamics that challenge social norms that re-enact exclusions and harm through racism, ableism, sanism, and transmisogyny. Thus, we reflect on the possibilities and problems of care at collective and community levels within trans and queer subcultures. We consider forms of care that seem generative and conducive for trans and queer lives, addressing a handful of practices that resonate with trans femmeness in particular. Collective and community care brim with possibilities – it can challenge the deep embedding of oppressions within one's body, unleashing potentials of embodied life: It can make life not only liveable, but joyous.

By care, we are speaking of the work and activities that attend to the physical and emotional needs of all life; this includes the skills and capacity of 'nurturing [...] all that is necessary for the welfare and flourishing of life'.[2] We find it useful to understand the *forms* care takes, for instance, mutual aid, therapy, care webs, emotional labour, social reproduction, or removing toxic environmental pollution, to look for different sorts of meaning that arise. Through these forms, we understand *practices* of care, for instance, getting groceries for another person who can't go to the shops, cooking or vacuuming or washing dishes, making space for difficult emotions with a friend, sharing resources, sending love when love is needed, and challenges in transitioning with others. There is not always a clear line between forms and practices of care, but thinking through the distinction allows for an understanding of *how* (in what form do) we come together and give meaning to our actions; while practices can speak of the concrete activities we undertake to mutually give and receive support from each other. Oftentimes people practise care without questioning the form in which this happens, which leaves questions about its meaning unattended. Linked to this comes another side of care, which we describe as attentiveness. This entails knowing

43

where your own attention goes and how one is sharing their attention with the world. Attention informs one's direction of actions and thereby delineates one's dependency on others to come to a fuller understanding of the world. It attends to questions of identification and separation. By identifying needs, desires and patterns of thought one is aware of what care can give, which skills need to be learnt, but also what one needs to unlearn – for instance, not daring to ask for care.[3] Nonnormative flourishing needs mutual attentiveness. We experience attentiveness as a necessary component of nurturing difference.

We also address what seems like care's flipside – harm. Our writing emerges from a place of having experienced (at times severe) harm, including from institutions. We describe below the significant differences between structural harm (e.g. regimes of economic austerity, institutional racism, or sexism) and accidental harm, but in all cases, harm calls for care as a reparative. Care supports dealing with the navigation of hostile social ecologies, whether they are institutional, social, or familial. Thus, we start this chapter from a premise of a dynamic between care and duress: how do we undo duress and where do we need care? In the dynamic between care and harm we find contemporary trans life. Neither care nor harm is evenly distributed over all trans life: positive attention is awarded to those of us who hover closer to the norms of whiteness and the middle-class, and forms of gendering that are recognised as more proper; negative attention is levied on those who are assumed to claim belonging, where others wish for this to be denied, which is co-constituted through racism, ableism, and xenophobia. Not all harm is the gory,[4] visible, and shocking scenes ending in death or mutilation, which are seemingly inevitable elements when trans lives are narrated. For instance, the scenes of harm displayed on days to commemorate lost trans lives (such as Trans Day of Remembrance) aren't necessarily experienced by those who attend these rituals in the Global North.[5] Some harm is medical in nature, such as the forced sterilisations that have been endured; some harm does not come across as harm, for instance, in the everyday contestations that wear one down.

While trans life is often displayed in narratives of harm, it is rarely shown as a form of flourishing. This is partly because contemporary neoliberal capitalism is not interested in flourishing, neither for trans life, nor for most other life. Care and attentiveness as forms of nurturing lead to flourishing – when they are not interrupted by duress. Thus, we elaborate care as an aspect of ethics that works to challenge the disposability and denigration of people marginalised by the dynamics of racism and anti-Blackness, trans- and queerphobia, class, ableism, sanism, and xenophobia. For us, this ethics is informed by femme sensibilities – which balance the practice and skills of care, the power and possibilities they forge, individually and in collectives; and the knowledge that femininity brings social expectations of care, with their attendant exploitation of our care skills.

HIERARCHIES OF CARE

As Leah Lakshmi Piepzna-Samarasinha writes, the expectation to perform care is tied into how femmes, and especially poor and/ or disabled and/or femmes of colour including sex workers, are valued in communities, which seemingly invites endless availability and work.[6] Care comes with an ingrained tension – caught between the demand to care for others and the need for care from each other – the problem seems to be the solution. However, this is a false conundrum that shows care is not the problem, but the lack of mutuality is. In hierarchies of care, to 'have to' care for another means to be obstructed in forming one's own life, while supporting someone else. In another words – when someone can do what they want, they might find themself in situations where others are taking care of their needs, within structures that allow their life to flourish. It is not for nothing that individualism is the hallmark of consumerist capitalism and managerial intervention: to impose their vision on the world without a care, or even assumed *as* care, is to find oneself up social hierarchies. In (professionalised or patriarchal) environments this means others are cleaning up after them, showing attentiveness, and in general letting go of personal needs in order to attend to theirs.

These hierarchies of care come with gendered and racialised dimensions. Overlooking the reproductive labour of Black, Brown, trans, queer, migrant, and other marginalised, feminised people entails enclosing oneself in a world of ease, itself rooted in extractive economies. These worlds play out in nuclear families, workplaces, care work, cleaning, and health care. In focusing on care, it is key to discern where agency is used, and to question whether care is the result of consent and negotiated responsibilities. This means in part that care can be demanded in the form of servitude, but can also take the form of collective resistance.

María Lugones confronts her own coming of age with a problem – the lack of identification with her mother and having 'grafted the substance of herself on her mother'.[7] This failure of identification does not only mean that she draws on the lifeforce of her mother to produce herself, but moreover that she lacks noting how her mother resists the demands placed upon her, and what gives her meaning in life. The gendered nature of this indifference does not run from a more traditional binary perspective man/woman, but mother/daughter. Lugones in the daughter role, rejected her mother's position as a child, but only later confronted herself with not finding ways to understand her mother's position, build solidarity, and question her own behaviour and attitudes. This returns in Lugones questions about who moves around with a certain ease in worlds, and how ethics can take shape based on this failure of identification.

Questioning affordances of living with ease reviews the direction of one's attention, agency, and mutuality in relations that are either marked by care or their lack of it. The ability to live with ease is unequally distributed, running through racialisations and gender. Who is afforded ease is ordered by institutionalised frameworks of social hierarchies, what Lugones might term the coloniality of gender.[8] Within social hierarchies the expectation is that care work is taken up by those that are 'marked out' for care: Black, Brown, migrant, femme, trans, queer, women. This is not simply achieved through oppression, precarity and wage labour, but also managed through absence of initiative, lack of communication, shrugging off responsibility, indifference and by enforced request.

These hierarchies and the resistance to them traverse the arguments that follow, with our proposal for mutuality of relations that is not predicated on affordance, ease, and indifference. Ethics is not about doing what you want, but ensuring that shared collectivity is at the heart of mutual relations. Having learnt that indifference produces hierarchies, and that hierarchical power relies on devalued care, we will discuss care as central to a transfeminist ethics, which undermines power structures and undoes separability. While demands for care increase a sense of responsibility, and individualism increases indifference, we are not just looking at care needs, but also attitudes and sensibilities that increase and broaden people's scope for ethics. We hope this chapter can contribute to a collective consciousness about our agency when it comes to caring, making relationalities and solidarity. Agency shapes actions that shift with cultural dynamics, age, gender and social status. Care ethics encourage us to unlearn disposability, while undoing the norms of gender, race and sexuality that devalue femmes.

CARE AND RIGHTS

From the context of neoliberal states in which we're writing, theorising, and living, rights are held up as a legitimate goal for liberation – amid denigration, harm, disposability, and carceral logics aimed at Black people, people of colour, migrants, disabled people, and poor people, and where LGBTQ people are overrepresented within economically precarious groups. The state and its institutions purport to provide legal and social structures, healthcare and welfare, yet become sites of distress, abuse, and violence for marginalised people. Their function is seemingly to support bodies and lives in the flow of norms (that may shift over time) of race, gender, ability, sexuality, religion, and citizenship, among others.[9] This was especially pronounced in 2020 during the COVID-19 pandemic, where epidemiological crisis was exacerbated by the failure of states to introduce effective virus containment measures, or to effectively protect people in care homes, or in prisons. In the context of state abandonment, many communities blossomed and were (re)made through mutual aid, providing support and learning skills to orient towards each other, reshaping social relations as we went.[10]

An awareness of institutional violence led us to understand that focusing on policy and rights does not serve our liberatory aims. Making ethics a basis for trans liberation, we ask how we might live our lives, and what we need in order to have a sense of futurity. This includes questioning how we relate to each other and what we attach meaning to, while relating to institutions with hesitancy. As abolitionists, we understand institutions are backed up by violence that will not protect people with needs that run counter to those institutions. Aligning with abolitionist politics encourages us to face each other no matter what, which includes facing our own, sometimes hard, emotions. In Chapters 1 and 3, we discuss these abolitionist ethics in terms of complicity and how it helps to structure solidarity. Here, we want to underline that abolition requires skills that are built up by creating spaces together – forging alternatives to relying on the powers that be. Given that we have no overarching structures of our own (such as the police) to call to protect our spaces, we find other ways of dealing with difficult situations.[11] Sometimes this means saying no, sometimes this means being very vocal about our yeses. Sometimes it means that we sit with each other to work through tough feelings, and attend to each other's bodily needs. Usually it entails learning to be generous and to *receive* care and support – to ensure the circle that we forge together doesn't break.

Capitalist society depends upon a racial and gendered division of labour, which, in the context of care, assigns the demands of care and waged care work disproportionately to 'feminised' bodies – where feminisation includes migrant, Black, Brown, and/or trans and queer bodies.[12] Some of us are recruited as low-paid and precarious care workers, making life liveable for others or reproducing private and public spaces. In our experience, LGBTQ+ people often find themselves working in the care sector.[13] Additionally, we may be disproportionately solicited to care for our families or households – whether we choose to undertake this work or not. The economic structure of care makes the family or 'the household' (which may be the site of the nuclear family, or its alternative) the primary domain of privatised care. Furthermore, neoliberal welfare reforms, including divestment and closure of services such as childcare, adult social care, and healthcare services, entail that the 'burden' of care labour weighs on the family or household, rather than costing the state.[14] The couple at the centre of the nuclear family can be hetero or homo, monogamous or not, although preferably affluent, able-bodied, and able to provide for the care of each other, their children or other dependents. The normative family may impose sexist support structures to reaffirm a masculine head. While masculinity is set up to receive collective support, those feminised are often made responsible for their own well-being. Thus, the disciplinary function of the family needn't be overt. In such forms, marginalised queer, trans, migrant, disabled, or Mad people may fall through the cracks of norms – although we may not all experience or feel this marginalisation.[15]

In turn, through care work, one may understand the demands of the racial and gendered division of labour at an embodied level. Feminised bodies disposable to capital's reproduction are often assumed to be disposed towards care (which can thus be exploited).[16] Or, as expendable bodies, if we refuse this work culture or are (physically, psychologically) unable to work by it, capital's devaluation of our bodies gets reinscribed into the dynamics of institutions. This may be discerned, for instance, in the reliance of middle-class families in the Global North on the labour of migrant workers from the Global South or Eastern Europe. Another example may be in institutional racism and sexism within large organisations, which reproduce racial and gendered pay gaps that disadvantage racialised and feminised workers. Such dynamics 'naturalise' the racial and gendered division of labour, reverberating into social reproduction. The racialised and gendered division of labour – in which some labour is devalued and some people are more worthy of success, care and comfort than others – gets writ large within our social contexts, through our own senses of self and each other. Redress through channels such as labour unions, and fighting for better working conditions, wages, resources, and space for precarious lives to exist, may challenge their harsh edges.

To suggest that *we are all worthy of care;* that *we can learn how to articulate and receive the care that we need;* and that *we may need to work less in order to focus on the care we all need to thrive* seem like radical claims in the context of twenty-first-century capitalist work culture grounded in overwork, overproduction, and scarcity. By focusing on everyday care, a politicised ethics may begin to combat capitalism's endless upward redistribution of wealth. Collective care practices solidarity in the face of disposability.

In addition, precarious material conditions mean that our collectives or communities don't have (access to) the same kinds of resources as the rich. Social exclusion means the hoarding of resources – such as land, wealth, time, leisure time, or access to education, or (physical or emotional) capacity. As the Care Collective writes in their 2020 *Care Manifesto*, 'both more time and adequate material resources are essential to ground and facilitate mutually fulfilling and imaginative practices of care, from the domestic to the planetary level.'[17] The need for adequate material resources – such as access to life-saving healthcare – ignited LGBTQ collective practices and politics over the last 50 years, and especially in regard to HIV/AIDS treatment and trans healthcare. Amid the lack of resources, we learn to make space for our needs, how to give care and how to care, acknowledging each other's boundaries. The practices of turning indifference to difference through care creates worlds, transforming alienation into connection.

Understanding care as giving form to the world together, dissolves the clear distinction between the caregiver and the care recipient. In its typical dichotomy, the caregiver is in a position of power (they may have legal guardianship; they might refuse to care) over the person receiving care. The care receiver is considered in need, and possibly misunderstood as lacking agency. This formulation might ignore the experiences of either person – supporting a narrative where the caregiver acts benevolently, and experiences no pleasure or satisfaction, while the care receiver doesn't have a choice in the matter. Such a general idea of charity regularly functions

as ableism by negating the agency of disabled people; and benevolent caregiving has a history rooted in white supremacy through
the gendered labour of bourgeois women (and white supremacist
practices of Christianity).[18] Hierarchical logics prioritise care for
one (at the expense of all); yet all forms of life need care, as decolonial, crip, posthumanist, queer, and trans thought, politics, and
practices argue.

AFFECTIVE ECONOMIES AND
THE DEVALUATION OF CARE

The devaluation and disposability of marginalised people is not
'merely cultural' – it impacts our social existences, our economic
opportunities, and our embodied lives. While marginalisation may
be overdetermined by one's position within social hierarchies and
one's identity, this is not the end of the story, nor does it provide
a strategy towards liberation. Here, we constellate a relationship
between how worthy any of us are of receiving the care we need (or
of being in relations of care more generally), and economics and
politics – including the forms of verbal and legal duress and support
that might be directed at marginalised people. We are mindful of
how worthy we/they are of living well; of being worked until physical
or psychological breakdown;[19] of health, justice, of rights within
neoliberal states, or of being incarcerated by them or removed from
them. Deconstructing these hierarchical relations and reflecting on
our complicity within them, a transfeminist ethics rooted in care
may (re)orient our actions towards change.

Queer theory has long been attuned to how political climates
influence our social worlds, including who we care *about* (delineated
from who we care *for* and *how*). The queer critique of homonationalism describes the role of emotions (or affect – the experience and
critical study of emotions) in (ethno)nationalist politics, which invite
citizens to passionately align themselves with the necropolitical or
necroliberal[20] nation-state – in contexts of Islamophobic, anti-mi-
grant, racist, and anti-trans rhetoric from representatives of the
state.[21] While homonationalism encompasses legal and economic

relations that enfold LGBTQ+ people into national belonging – through gay marriage, freedom to be out in the military, and hate crime protections – this critique describes how *the circulation of feelings* maintains social divisions (separability). The 'circulation and mobilization of feelings of desire, pleasure, fear, and repulsion utilised to seduce all of us into the fold of the state' is described as an 'affective economy' by Anna Agathangelou, Morgan Bassichis, and Tamara Spira (following Julia Sudbury), naming 'the various ways in which we become invested emotionally, libidinally, and erotically in global capitalism's mirages of safety and inclusion'.[22] Moreover, this entails 'naturaliz[ing] [...] who truly belong[s] in the grasp of state captivity', through incarceration and policing, destruction and death via war, domestically and internationally.[23]

Elsewhere, Sara Ahmed uses affective economies to describe how affects (such as hate and fear) accrue meaning through their movement between objects and signs, which – in the case of fear – 're-establishes distance between bodies whose difference is read off the surface'.[24] For instance, the activation of fear in proximity to racialised bodies is 'crucial to establishing the "apartness" of white bodies'.[25] Re-reading a famous scene in Frantz Fanon's *Black Skins, White Masks* – of the emotional upheaval of the white child encountering the Black man – Ahmed elaborates how the emotional drama of the scene is *about* the feelings of the white child, as the child mis/reads the response of a Black man, who is in turn constructed as Other through the scene. Anti-Black and racist responses to the presence of Black, Indigenous, or brown people emerge in the context of the histories, structural foundations, and socialities of racial capitalism that link to settler colonialism, the transatlantic slave trade, plantation economies, colonial monopolies, indentured labour, and empires and their reconstructions after formal decolonisation. Gender in excess of the colonial sex/gender binary – as a modality of radical resistance, and as subject of coloniser's contempt – has been in the mix of these historical processes, as trans of colour theorists C. Riley Snorton, Tourmaline, and Marquis Bey remind us.[26]

Today, conversations involving transphobic feminists (or apologists for settler colonialism for that matter), often come to be about the victimisation felt by those in dominant positions. The actual needs, experiences, harms, and material struggles of those marginalised by domination fall out of view. For instance, in February 2024, former UK Prime Minister Rishi Sunak made transphobic comments during Prime Minister's Questions, while the Mother of Brianna Ghey, a trans teenager murdered in a transphobic attack, was in the House. The act of transphobic homocide and the cultural context within which Brianna's murder occurred, alongside the community grief felt from it, are only 'addressed' by the reaffirmation of transphobia, rather than any recognition of this violence, its impact, and the need for solidarity and support. Transfeminism conceptualises the everyday dynamics of disavowal and denigration of our thought, our work or labour, our affects and needs, which constitute transmisogyny, transphobia, and the specific hatred aimed at gender non-conforming people.[27]

The cultural and the economic are deeply co-constituted – social attitudes are interrelated with the racial and gender divisions of labour that tries to (over)determine the value of our labour power (and of our work more broadly), and how it feels to exist in our particular bodyminds. Rosemary Hennessy describes the inseparability of affect, culture and capital/ism through the formulation of a 'second skin'.[28] Emphasising how it feels to be in, to feel through, one's skin, Hennessy describes a second skin as 'a tissue of values that organizes sensations and affective intensities'.[29] These values are the cultural values that ground how we understand ourselves, map our bodies and feel through our flesh, by the way of norms, representations, discourses, histories, subcultures, and more. They are 'open' as 'sites of struggle', as moments of harm and resistance in the wider public sphere may be felt through this sensory organ. But they are also open to capital: racial and gendered divisions of labour proscribe opportunities of workers and also the possibilities of one's life – these divisions (re)produce *social* abjection. Through ethnographic accounts of *maquiladora* workers on the Mexican *frontera*, Hennessy describes how homophobia, transphobia and misogyny work in concert to denigrate queer workers, deny them social protections, and pay them less.[30] On the flipside, labour struggles and legal battles for employment protections to support LGBTQI+, disabled, racialised, and migrant workers, directly push back against capital's devaluations. Second skins orient a compass of how it feels to be in our ensouled bodyminds at a given hirstorical moment, amid the currents undergirding our social worlds.

The two formulations of affective economies emphasise the role emotions play in cohering national(ist) citizen-subjects into cultural norms, engineering distance and social division – or *separability*[31] – between those who belong according to these norms and those who are actively excluded by them. Hennessy's second skins conceptualise the trials, harms, and struggles that get written on the surface of workers' bodies, as cultural politics and social life permeate the workplace. The belonging with, or abjection from, norms mapped by affective economies influence the value of one's second skin, while, amid climates of hostility, we navigate our work days. It would be deeply naïve to suggest that the political climate – of national belonging manufactured through imaginaries that stir hatred and fear – does not influence our social relations, including our care relations. In the context of our formulation of complicity, it is urgent that we reflect on the reproduction of separability through our actions and through how our social lives are organised. How do we orient our practices to dissolve the exclusions of these arrangements? How do we work through the complicities that align our affects – our pleasures and repulsions – and our social worlds and relations, with dynamics of separability? What about in institutional relations and bureaucracy, which we may assist in reproducing and upholding? (We discuss this in the next chapter.) In this climate of hostility, practices of collective and community care can intervene in the processes of belonging and abjection, of value and denigration, including the economic devaluation of care work, to enact different forms of affective economy.

Care entails life-giving and sustaining activities, an absence of which may entail abandonment into abjection, or towards (slow) death.[32] Care ethics proposes a materialism to make bodyminds and lives come to 'matter' in the sense of social and cultural worth. It brings into focus activities of care work to counter transphobic or transmisogynist or xenophobic or racist denigrations. These are concrete interactions with living beings or the spaces we inhabit, rather than simple statements of 'care' or solidarity.[33] Thinking reflectively about our care practices in relation to separability, we can consider who is with us in these moments, and who is missing, of enacting or receiving care. We typically provide or receive care within classed, racialised, familial, or institutional or community-oriented settings; or we are employed or solicited to provide/receive (paid) care work (potentially) across these lines. (Collective care may create forms that are an exception, or partly an exception.) In addition, as Sophie Lewis argues, typical kinship is often inadequate for meeting our desires for care, especially in the contexts of home-lessness and precarity, histories of (ongoing) settler colonialism, and of transphobic, queerphobic and sexist violence.[34] Thinking through care and abolition helps to bridge structural divides, even if those divides aren't completely overcome in the process.

Our ethical orientations can both reproduce and counter separa-bility, reproducing, and/or dissolving the order of racial capitalism (in local, or direct, ways). Materialism, Marxism, and Marxist feminism emphasise the importance of our actions in the world – the transformations they produce, the norms they reproduce – even when they are without economic value, or seem unimportant in the context of capitalist norms. After all, neoliberalism wouldn't hold up if we didn't obey its commands, some of which are imperative, some moral – hence, the power in the idea to 'become ungovernable'.[35] In discussing complicity and femmeness, we acknowledge that all of us get tied into neoliberal expectations – but thinking care through femmeness encourages looking out for each other in these contexts, and registering how these expectations divert our actions away from the things, people or worlds that nourish and shape our lives. In its multiplicities, care *is a resource that we can reorientate towards sup-porting our worlds, our friends, our lovers, and even passing strangers, to exist and thrive.* It is one tool to challenge the disposability of marginalised people, to undo stigmas that deem some people more worthy of life than others. The ethos of prison abolition proposes that no one is disposable; practices of care nourish life in the face of disposability. We are conscious of the need to move beyond practices focused on survival, and towards interconnected care practices for humans and non-humans, working towards our collective flourishing. Good care can be the ground for exploring desires and growing worlds, nourished by love and budding with possibility. Our actions manifest possibilities of social transformation by tending the social contra capitalism.

FORMS OF CARE

As precarious trans and queer femmes, it is in and through practices of care that we've healed and been held; that we've experienced love (personal and social); and in care's absence found ourselves nursing bruises and scars. Some of these scars speak of traumas past and present, of hurt from the institutions we have been raised through (schools, the family), but also from within the queer and trans communities that felt like home. At the time of writing, care, as a concept, has been in vogue, although in speaking from marginalised perspective intones its qualities and its necessity differently. It is from and with disabled and Mad, queer, and trans and 2SQ, Black, Indigenous, of colour, white, and/or migrant people that we have studied care and practised it in our everyday lives.[36] This is no coincidence – it's from within social struggles that we delve deeper into what our needs look like, how they may be met outside of the given institutions of life under capitalism – in the knowledge that these processes of exploration and vulnerability might shape friendships and relationships, collectives and communities, and the (sub)cultures and worlds that emerge through them. In this section, we delineate *forms* of care that have emerged through theory and popular discourses, rooted in collective social struggles which work(ed) to address immediate needs.

Focusing on one's personal needs, especially when we've been taught that they don't matter and that someone else's are more important, is one way to recognise the shape of one's world. To develop and come to an understanding of one's needs in political and collective contexts, where one comes to articulate them among people who may share those needs, opens up these emotional and embodied developments. However, it's not easy – as Leah Lakshmi Piepzna-Samarasinha writes of 'crip emotional intelligence', as an important skill understood through disability justice frameworks, it entails 'knowing you will probably have to offer help a million times before another disabled person takes you up on it'.[37] Part of the work of overcoming oppressions, including internalised oppressions, entails countering the voices and affective economies that claim we are not worthy of support, while building the social infrastructures and worlds that can open the space to articulate one's needs – in a way that is couched in consent.

Care may often take the form of social reproductive labour, theorised by Marxist feminists to describe how the care work necessary for the maintenance of life on a daily basis creates labour power – the labour that (re)produces capital, institutions and public and private spaces. This includes activities that have been historically understood as 'feminised' labour, such as cooking and feeding, birthing and rearing children, housework and laundry, and sex work. Recent writings on family abolition show how the privatisation of labour around sexual and social reproduction within 'the' (nuclear) family is increasingly unsustainable for many involved, operating through fictions of belonging manufactured through 'family values'.[38] The International Wages for Housework movement, across the 1970s and 1980s, challenged the naturalisation of unpaid housework as labour by arguing its centrality to the capitalist economy and demanding remuneration.[39] Marxist feminists argue that this care work is feminised by a hierarchical racial and gendered division of labour (discussed above), where structural social and economic forces lead to certain jobs being commonly worked by individuals of a particular gender, race, sexuality, or migration history.[40] Elsewhere, Nat has written about the particularities of social reproduction for queer and trans life, that the labour and care work that ensures queer and trans people continue to exist entails different practices, amid conditions of precarity and social abjection. She argues for the need to expand the concept of social reproduction through centring queer and trans folks, making legible the caring, affective and gender labor that enables and maintains queer and trans bodies and lives – the loving and sexual pleasure, cooking and feeding and housing, resting and rearing, cleaning and washing and dressing, the emotional and psychological support, transition support, healthcare support, the work of creating our performative genders and gender expressions, the very fabrication of us.[41]

The practices of care that nurture and cohere around trans and queer bodies have often themselves been ignored, dismissed, or misunderstood – these practices are essential to our survival and everyday existence. Nat discusses how queer and trans domesticity may take alternative forms to those of social norms, such as those enacted by Street Transvestite Action Revolutionaries with STAR House, NYC, in the 1970s, where homeless sex worker trans and gay youth, predominantly people of colour, made a home together and supported each other; and that the acts of care we may need to heal (in various ways) involve understanding our particularities. The embodied experiences that come with marginalisation, and in addition the kinds of care that trans and non-binary people may seek to transform our lives and our bodies, vary from norms – in terms of how we seek them, who provides them, and how they affectively refigure our being.

One form of care that has reached common parlance in recent years is emotional labour. This describes the capacity that holds space for affective validation, exploration and expression, primarily in others (although not exclusively); it entails buffering and acknowledging experiences, including those that are harmful. Practising attentiveness, actively listening, which we discuss at length below, both entail emotional labour. Hence, emotional labour is not simply 'immaterial' – it is a key aspect of practice which maintains social life and social justice organising: 'Manage logistics, answer feelings emails, show up, empathise, build, and maintain relationships. Organize the childcare, the access support, the food. Be screamed at, de-escalate, conflict resolute'.[42] To be good at providing emotional labour does require skill, skills which may be born from personal experiences, including of distress. Because emotional labour is undervalued as skill and practice, it is unequally demanded and distributed according to social hierarchies – as Leah Lakshmi details in their 'Modest Proposal for a Fair Trade Emotional Labour Economy'.[43] Marginalisation breeds social isolation when one doesn't have anyone to lean on for emotional support themselves. The skills that are grown through emotional labour can be set to work to build worlds. This might entail adjusting organisational structures and distributing attention to ensure that those marginalised receive their due. Sometimes, this comes with protecting a space for pleasure that would otherwise be invaded by affects, demands, tensions, trauma, difficulty and negativity. Spaces of recuperation are needed after the intensities of labour and/or struggle, or after we have experienced harm.

One such form of space is the queer social structure of chosen family. Born out of the abjection that many queer and trans people face in the normative family, chosen families challenge its consolidation of care. Chosen family is borne out of intentional kinship and support out of necessity and/or fun; they may be forged in a context of migration, and not explicitly labelled as 'family' from the outset. The 'fam' may encompass a multitude of relational forms – chosen siblings, intergenerational parenting (that may not be defined by age difference), and sometimes sexual relationships. These relations may be defined through shared experience, or in guiding someone through shared or similar experiences. Chosen families pool skills, knowledge, and resources – practical ones as well as those (inextricable) from care; they are spaces of reprieve, love, learning, and growth, of emotional labour towards support and uplift. At best, this may be unconditional; although togetherness and support might be temporally bound, helping marginalised people navigate particularly challenging or transformative periods in our lives. Chosen families may focus on the domestic space, and in that sense may reproduce gendered norms.

CARE IN COLLECTIVE LIFE

In the context of our analysis, we delineate collective care and broader community care, and some of the forms they take within trans and queer, disability justice, and feminist subcultures. Collective care describes self-organised, direct, and focused forms of support – which may be practical, emotional, medical, or otherwise. Collective care attends to needs while remaining oriented to a world – what a group of us need on a daily basis to live, heal, rest, or work, or potentially thrive, and how can these care needs be met (in what form, and by whom). Collective care encourages us to come to understand what our needs are – to ask ourselves *how* we are struggling with living, or what might we need for our lives to bear fruit. Understanding our own needs is itself a skill that institutionalised contexts may suppress, and that capitalism encourages us to displace or offset through consumption. As A.J. Withers describes, understanding and articulating one's care needs – even as a disabled queer activist and writer – can be challenging, as one fights internalised oppressions (such as ableism) and one's devaluation as a person and bodymind worthy of care, which may be rooted deep within oneself.[44] We understand collective care as involving direct interactions, often intimacy and friendship, making oneself vulnerable in the exposition of one's needs. This is not one-directional – vulnerability might, for instance, leave one open to disrespect and harm if one's needs are dismissed; but practising vulnerability can encourage others to show up beyond individual initiative. Vulnerability reveals its power in mutuality.

Collective care might describe a care team that comes over to check in on you when you're stuck at home for whatever reason, brings you food or does your dishes when you're in need of support, and helps you go to the bathroom when you're not able to on your own. It's organising the care web that supports you when you're just out of hospital, after a major surgery or injury, or in the everyday of high needs. In such reparative forms, collective care functions at the level of social reproduction, ensuring on a daily basis that one is able to do what one needs to live. In practice, a care collective may be organised on an online spreadsheet or Google Doc, communicating via group chat or WhatsApp or Signal Messenger, checking in on capacity in the group, putting out requests to run errands or crossing them off the list when they're completed. This collective may include your friends, housemates, friends of friends, or paid personal assistants – although we would like to emphasise that support is provided because people care about your existence in the world; indeed, a lack of this care may feel like, as Withers describes, cracks in one's universe.[45] Compared to institutional care (including that of the family), collective care encourages the flattening of hierarchies. Within this care ethics, one is motivated to do care work, even if this motivation is also economic. But without nourishment and support, carers may burn out or disappear.

Furthermore, collective care can overcome the isolation or lack of support that many marginalised people face. However, there is a double bind, as isolation by definition is a lack of the people one needs or desires to make worlds with. As Leah Lakshmi discusses, any individual's care shouldn't have to depend on popularity or worthiness; however, the norms of affective economies are commonplace, and communities and collectives can reproduce ableism, sanism, whiteness, racism, and anti-Blackness, femmephobia, queerphobia, and transmisogyny, as social credit and satisfying activities follow existing hierarchies.[46] These feelings can indicate an expectation of who is caring for whom; or of having time to care for one, while feeling or being unable to care for another. Such dynamics in dominant groups and normative contexts marginalise of our needs. Thus, collective care necessitates unlearning social norms that bolster white cis-hetero-abled-patriarchal dynamics, that dismiss the rest of us as unworthy. Expressing marginalised needs may reveal 'hidden' dynamics of exploitation and neglect, while encouraging active learning. We need to hold space for the hurt that comes with this social organisation of neglect, and leverage this hurt and the ambivalence of care work against neoliberal, racial capitalism.[47]

Care collectives often emerge out of marginalised communities or subcultures. Communities themselves cohere through care and may provide care to those within and outside of them. Care itself is an essential element *in* collective organising for liberatory aims, in order to function and facilitate space for each other in the group. It entails reading the affective and work dynamics at play, supporting each other within those dynamics. This is, however, not about *managing* or suppressing emotional differences, particularly in the case of interpersonal conflict or the reproduction of harmful social norms. Collective contexts where care is *not* practised may lead to burnout, abuse of power and harm.

HARM AND GENDER DYNAMICS

In considering care and attentiveness from a femme perspective, we do not equate care and positionality, nor think that care is something femmes are inclined to do or do better than others – even if care is solicited *from* us. Care is necessary in maintaining non-exploitative relations with people, alongside non-human life and ecosystems. These connections are held by attentiveness and practices that develop through consent and can be learnt by most. Other versions of feminist ethics of care, for instance, that put forward by Nel Noddings, made claims that placed care firmly with some genders more than others.[48] Noddings proposed that some genders come with an ethics that is not masculine, institutional and rule-based, but instead care, because these genders were more aware of vulnerabilities. This ethics rightly (in our eyes) received criticism about enshrining care to a specific gender, re-inscribing gendered expectations of who ought to be providing care in an essentialist manner. This is not our position, as it is unclear how it leads to liberation.

Neoliberal society forces us to care by relying on sexism to maintain socially reproductive labour. We find that gendered exploitation is possible through the counterpoint to care – that is, indifference, an attitude that separates people into an affective hierarchy. We see this indifference as the result of extractivism founded in the colonial dispossession of Indigenous people, and other humans and animals from their lands in order to exploit these lands, humans (including through chattel slavery and indenture, but also through some contemporary practices of wage labour), and animals as resources. Neglect, abuse, and murder are necessary for colonialism. The hierarchical attitudes of extractivism operate through affects us in our everyday lives, because such attitudes rub off into social life. How one is (up)held through the norms of racial capitalism is what we need to attend to, towards undoing this hierarchy. In addition, trans femme life has taught us about disposability. It is what we face when, having spoken up in communities or collectives, one finds oneself isolated; or when one voices necessary accommodations in a relationship or a workplace, one gets dumped or is made redundant; or when one finds oneself alone in a moment of crisis. At the same time, countering disposability and hegemony in affective economies involves building deep connections, attentiveness, and love. The intimate and social structure of gender informs our approach to the role of care in an ethics of making worlds that run counter to institutionalised indifference.

We think of harm as the interruption of living by violence. Harm at the individual level shrinks chances at life. Harm occurs when violence interrupts one, regardless of your interactions with the world. This can be the violence of social hierarchies and their alienation; the structural violence reproduced in domestic spaces by partners, family, parents; the violence that lurks in our communities because people ride rough-shod over other people's life experiences.[49] Relatedly, duress is the structural form social power takes, but duress does not always lead to harm – either because we are protected by each other, or by practices of care, support and solidarity that interrupt hegemonic narratives, and so on. Laura Ann Stoler discusses duress as the longitudinal effect of colonialism that contains life in shrunken potentialities, violence, and harshness. While duress can show up as harm, duress can also be understood as the absence of options, such as in the violent enclosures of prisons, but also in a lack of possibilities in life – including of liberation.[50] This can also take the form of violence of debt, poverty, precarity that keeps people stressed, on their toes, or immiserated; the structural violence of the police, social workers, and civil servants levied against the poor; the structural violence of Stop and Search, arrests, imprisonment; the domestic abuse that takes the form of beatings, criticism, denial of needs, denial of perspective; the propagandistic violence that beats down from right-wing, xenophobic media, the endless stream of transphobic columns in righteous left-wing newspapers; the administrative violence of proving gender, holding gendering norms up to binary categories; the fight for medical attention, medical care, or housing to recuperate from all this. While violence leads to harm, too often duress is turned in on itself, and takes the shape of everyday indifference and ignorance. Duress is partly the result of an alienated epistemology, that cannot connect to those it has marginalised. This makes it, at times, merely a fact of life that has to be navigated. These structures do not necessarily harm, they can be lampooned, be so recognisable that they are futile, or are so commonplace that they do not touch one – even if they block 'moving up the ranks'.

A politics of anti-harassment that leans on a gendered division of aggression-versus-care indirectly draws upon bourgeois virtuousness. When proper behaviour is the solution, rather than consent and activating collectivity, the institution of a new normativity is at stake. We're not looking for a politics of innocence and modesty, because relying on people being virtuous is not liberating, and evades social organising. The social relations of our care ethics are fundamental to drawing care out of the neoliberal quagmire of individual responsibility. Emphasising its social side leads to a form of humility regarding one's epistemic and agential reach, that undergirds the interdependence of collective work. Conversely, individual virtuousness relies on institutional processes and correctly fitting into a group by embodying norms – it homogenises social hierarchies, and not everyone's virtue is measured in the same way. A politics that takes this shape is dangerous for people that are racialised and/or trans and queer, because of the perils of hypervisibility with its connected paranoid epistemologies that attribute bad intentions.[51] Individual virtuousness undergirds white fragility, where the worst that can happen is to do bad and thus be bad, called out and cancelled.[52] Here, an approach that starts with 'you're doing it wrong' transposes into 'you are wrong', which structures disposability and abandonment, and struts up managerial attitudes. It leads to a sociality of not wanting to be seen with the wrong crowd. These processes make evident why relying on shifting forms of participation is necessary: as we are neither a single I, nor a homogenous 'we'.

While morality is based on alignment with institutions and behaving correctly,[53] ethics looks at the patterns that make us who we are and that we want to hold, regardless of the interruptions the world presents – whether these are structural or bad luck.[54] Ethics entails finding a way to live already in a post-capitalist future. Living in such a way requires building skills of relation – technes – that can withstand interruptions by violence, history, trauma, poverty, and precarity, or domestic abuse. This means building a world of knowledge and practices that help us through the present. The emergence of abolitionist politics and practices into the mainstream after the 2020 Black Lives Matter uprisings and protests following the murder of George Floyd are a testament to this. Abolitionist ethics then, does not focus on 'winning' against the capitalists or the state. If we look at the history of rebellion and uprisings in that manner, as Françoise Vergès reminds us by way of E.P. Thompson, we face a history of defeats.[55] Instead, we *read* a long line of rebellions that give us insights, tactics, strategies, outcomes, and ways of maintaining ourselves, despite the range of aggression that has been levied at us or even enacted by us.

In theorising the role of complicity through an abolitionist ethics, we find it important to question the dichotomy of victims and perpetrators. Victims do not get to occupy the space of innocence versus the perpetrator who needs to be cast out. Neither do we, as trans femmes, speak solely from a perspective of disposability, or from a position untouched by social power where we cannot do harm. Each one of us is variously implicated in the wrongs of this world, with social situations that have gone astray, relationships gone bad, situations that have been taken out of our hands, and our names used for punishing people. These things sometimes seem inevitable. Sometimes harm seems inevitable because we didn't learn to take care of ourselves and give a better direction to situations. At other times, situations went wrong because we couldn't support our communities; or they went wrong because we had to learn nuances about oppression and trauma. However, reflecting insights regarding different contexts through complicity can enable thinking and considering how things could have gone another way.[56]

A transfeminist ethics oriented towards futures relies on bonding – over interests, collaborations, care, pleasure, awareness of harm received, or transmitted; it builds and maintains communal life through connections of identity, or across groups or geographies. Refusing to remain static, this ethics holds space for the plural worlds that we live in,[57] the commitments that we live by, and the care and attention that we deserve to share.

SOCIAL LIFE: EMBODIED ATTENTIVENESS
AGAINST HEGEMONIC NORMS

Neoliberals love talking about community, and yet neoliberal policy will also do anything to rupture actual community – in order to redistribute power and resources upwards (thereby stabilising hegemonic logics), while invoking ideologies that make communities responsible for making up the loss that redistribution inflicted upon them.[58] This also entails the extraction of care, where care, for instance for diversity, may be demanded from an individual(ised) worker by the institution. While institutions support indifference, depositing problems out of sight and claiming that alternatives are 'unrealistic' or 'not our job', care ethics encourages that we turn towards and attend to frictions in the world.

In the forms of care and communities that are forged to counter neoliberal duress, whether they are friend groups, lovers, ex-partners, partners, acquaintances, visitors, or paid carers, we experience connection as well as friction. We care because we need and desire it, but our argument is that caring leads to a better form of life, where people can flourish. As Elizabeth Povinelli teaches us, 'to care is to embody an argument about what a good life is and how such a good life comes into being'.[59] For Povinelli, it is not about who cares more or who cares less, but that the form care takes is a proposition for the form of this world. Care can become dominating, even surveillance, when it doesn't leave room for differences.[60] Care is constraining when it demands to adhere to codes, because it imposes normativity on the practical truths that we learnt by navigating the world.

However, Povinelli indicates why an embodied approach to care can hold potentiality in a realistic way.

Looking at care in this way shows why the emergence of forms of life is inescapable. Embodiment contains propositions for potential futures and modes of flourishing. The 'emergency exit' that was promised by previous philosophies of indeterminacy (from Gilles Deleuze to Michael Warner) is therefore only a partial view that pulls the break on an entrenched passage into the future – it can become in Marquis Bey's words 'an anarchic sashay into the unknown'.[61] However, a focus on indeterminacy leads to stagnancy, because it cannot embody other modes of sociality. It is through embodied care that something else will be brought into the world. Care is a localised form of shaping futurity in trans femme worldings. And as such it is a contextual exploration and interrogation of the futures we want to live. These forms of living that are grown in practice are necessarily limited because the renegotiation of relations can only go so far.

Forms of life grow by giving them attention. This care for the world is also structured by concepts, attentiveness, and how it makes space for differences and openness. The materiality of ideas and experience-informed concepts underline that care alone is not enough. Attention to shifting practices explores how to make space for new forms of life and collective living, and in doing so, finds new ways to dismantle hegemony and duress. Change is not a replacement of the old for the new in a capitalist cycle, where all logics stay the same while discerning what to grow and what to decompose. Transformative explorations of survival and flourishing require new concepts to open new modes of connection and relation. New concepts are, for instance, held by the stories we tell, the poetics we lean on, the logics we apply, and the rhythms and patterns subtending our lives. When we interrogate, explore, and play we are making new concepts and forms. Attentiveness and care ensure making new forms of living is not a bootstrapping exercise – but pulling each other up and towards different ways of engagement. Theory is not ahead of practice.

One of the propositions of normativity that we critique in this book is that inattentiveness is due to 'ignorance', or a lack of knowledge. The idea that knowledge is sufficient for liberation is untrue. It follows a capitalist investment in futurity where a lack needs to be filled in order for everything to be ok. Ignorance is a structure of indifference that enables exploitation.[62] Growing out of indifference requires a different form of ethics. Forming the right relations needs time – this emphasis in ethics is termed *techne*. As Elizabeth Povinelli suggests, relational skills contain propositions for social forms because they attend to the world; and in that sense, they function like care, and indeed with care, proposing a manner of flourishing.[63] We want to underline that *any* form of relating is a relational skill: from liberatory care work, to also socialised indifference and alienation that enforce hierarchy at the cost of connection. Any relation thus contains a proposition for the form of the world, transformative *or* normative.

This means that anybody can contribute to transformative change. Indeed, we need everybody for liberation and that is not going to be easy (partly because we might need to recognise that people, including ourselves, need to be liberated from assumptions that we hold dear). Fast-forwarding the hope for liberation by projecting hopeful claims onto currently existing forms of social organisation, might not support flourishing but in fact do the opposite. For instance, modes of institutional behaviour, like individualism, make us worse off.[64] Whatever knowledge we hold, however many books we read, and how well we listen will not necessarily change the disruptive patterns generated by hegemonic modes of social organisation. What we need are different modes of relation, structured through different ways of knowing the world. To change that is why we listen, why we read, and why we act differently.

ATTENTIVENESS, SKILLS, CONSENT
AND ACCOUNTABILITY

In this last section, we will discuss some of the care that goes into making relationships that can strengthen social movements, by attending to difficult moments that occur, like abuse, hierarchies, and extraction. This includes the situating and developing the role of consent in social transformation. Care in its multidimensionality draws on a range of resources: embodied sense, thought, emotions, analysis, and skills of learning and relating, i.e. techne. Care is a form of *somatechnics* – the embodied modes of relationality that come with forms of knowing, feeling, and sensing the world.[65] Care is situated and requires developing very different aspects of oneself. For instance, we might have been taught to care about institutions more than about the people in them. We might have been taught that gender involves an unequal distribution of care, where whiteness, masculinity, and ability underline worthiness of attention, and femininisation and racialisation entail having to provide that attention. On another level, we may have been taught that to be correct is more important than to make space, as is a common problem on the left. Care thus also involves paying attention to what we need to unlearn.

One particular techne of care is attentiveness – which can assist in keeping one engaged in a world, or in detangling mixed-up understanding and issues. This includes recognising when our understanding falls back in binaries of 'good and bad', and considering what kind of engagement is warranted in a particular situation. For instance, sometimes we may excuse people with a certain bias because they do not know better, but that doesn't mean they need to be tolerated. Another example would be that, in caring for the environment, we might lock ourselves to runways, which shows courage and care; although the care shown in that regard is no substitute for care in interpersonal relationships, which cannot be traded off.

Furthermore, attentiveness involves acknowledging those who refuse. When in collectives the possibility to say 'no' is ignored, the people who need to say no most often end up isolated. Pluralist movements nurture the conditions of saying 'no', together with 'yes and ...', in action. Although saying 'yes' is not unequivocally easy – in mixed collectives, this means unlearning social hierarchies and learning the craft of holding on across difference and conflict. These skills can be built on spiritual commitments, social needs, wisdom, love, and relational ties, in addition to being understood as forms of labour.[66] However, when the maintenance of relations becomes one-sided, it becomes labour. Exploitation depends on unequal attention to relations – and those of us lower in the hierarchy are made responsible for the emotional work of maintenance. Those who avoid developing relational crafts are rarely confronted. A proverbial situation is when white, cis, straight men are 'emotionally unavailable', avoiding responsibility for relations. It creates an imbalance that demands care, and shapes a closed loop: what is often termed 'privilege' is an expectation that the world bends to one's needs.[67] This also means that some 'privileged' actors end up with only a small set of relational skills, which reinforces normative affective economies. So, a lack of relational skills creates a reliance on social power, which is used to extract care and attention from others to maintain its relations. Meanwhile, the refusal to bend to power can also be understood as a demand that such 'privileged' actors develop their relational skills.[68] 'Privileged' actors may otherwise remain ignorant of their limited relational skills because these skills are crafted through participation in the forms of relating where hierarchies do not hold.

Consent depends on a deep understanding of social positions and structures of relation and attentiveness.[69] Awareness of embodied perspectives and social structures is necessary for movements to maintain pluralities. Practising consent to support different ways of worlding is underrated, compared to knowing about oppression. The emphasis on knowing about oppression can lead to *disem*bodied approaches, which ignore the practices that sustain social hierarchies.[70] Again, ignoring practices creates a reliance on 'no' from people and avoids the care necessary to shape new ways of making space. In this sense, practising consent supports learning non-hierarchical approaches to sharing space. Underlining consent as a practice of actively looking for a 'yes' (in all its different forms) in combination with accountability invites curiosity about the way worlds are made. Care and consent are key to making space for joy, by looking at actions (and not just speech acts). Conversely, the need to walk out, often because it is the only possibility, can leave trans femmes alone or consign us to the internet, sometimes without the possibility of developing the relational styles we desire, retreating into worlds of feeling that are disconnected from lived entanglements. And yet, these speculative worlds are powerful in the sense that they can highlight what makes a different world and which elements it could lean on, which we will talk about in Chapter 5.

Another example of how attentiveness facilitates the development of new relational skills is found in Mariame Kaba's insightful discussion about rape in social movements. Kaba observes with nuance how sexual violence gets covered up with the demand for a tough solution.[71] It is challenging to bring nuance into an environment that is structured by disembodied knowledge and categorical thinking. For instance, crass discussions on social media are not helpful for building collectives.[72] In collectives a lot of work needs to be put into encouraging vulnerability to such an extent that people want to become accountable.[73] Kaba reminds us that accountability cannot be forced upon people, but is something that comes out of a desire or will to change. Making spaces to get together and feel free is a key element of social transformation.[74] Yet, social transformation comes with interpersonal conflicts. In these situations, we see the use of victimisation to avoid accountability.[75] We put our hurts on display to avoid having to explain our actions. Mariame Kaba reflects that accountability is not fun or even healing – even if it might be the first step towards healing.[76] Jay Bernard muses on how being called to account makes us feel degraded, perhaps even policed.[77] It is not easy to face each other and ourselves, to remain open and feel our fractures, and to feel that we can be in spaces where we can share what's going on. Sometimes we seem to prefer living side by side because living face to face can feel too much like confrontation. Doing things together may involve confrontation and frustration, amidst which all our personal problems can surface. How can we embrace anger from our communities, our friends, our accomplices and allies as a force that nonetheless helps us move together in a direction towards new forms of living? When we fuck up, some of us are given more leeway than others, get a second chance, or a third, or are never called to account. On the left, we think about power *over* us, not about power *in* our spaces. Problems in our spaces turn all too quickly into bourgeois morality plays that stage virtuousness and translate friction into 'acceptable' misunderstandings, rather than accountability.

Even when thinking through care, methods of making things right are not always clear-cut. It takes time to learn how to make amends to those we have harmed. We might need to build a collective structure that protects people against repetitions of harm; or the actions of one collective member may make it difficult to trust the whole group. Individualising the problem does not address the context that allowed harm to emerge. Transforming a space requires the commitment of all participants within it, but people can and do also leave. Plodding on, we strategise how to respond to situations – that get stuck rather than leading to transformation. We fret about the commitment we can offer. In lefty spaces, at the time of writing, there's consensus that policing is not acceptable; meanwhile, people utilise therapeutic language to push each other around.[78] Middle-class solutions are usually arranged with reference to the police or to therapy, and new norms may be adopted without critical reflection.[79] Therapy can be a life-saver, but whether therapeutic concepts can be deployed to solve tensions in social spaces is another question. Having refused to resort to the violence associated with the police, and given that, as we noted at the start, accountability does not bring healing *per se*, we need either strong, deep commitments to a collective or community, or we have to face up to really limited alternative options. Mariame Kaba states that while 'abolition is not about your feelings', dealing with feelings while trying to transform spaces seems inevitable.[80] As Kaba explains, transformative justice as a local practice that is not just a replacement or stand-in for criminal justice requires shifting group interactions, which comes with emotional upheaval. 'Accountability processes often feel terrible for people while they are in it'.[81] What is at stake, for Kaba, is that a survivor of harm gets to reclaim their agency, rather than needing to be treated as if they are fragile.[82] So, while accountability needs to start with a (collective) openness to accepting responsibility for actions and commitments, its results restore agency.

SHIFTING SENSES AS TRANS FORMATION

We close this chapter with a final note on attentiveness, on care and trans embodiment. One of the pleasures of trans theory is the possibility of feeling differently. Let's linger a little longer on Eva Hayward's note on transness as being 'sensorily redone'.[83] Hayward's comment that '[h]ormones, in this way, are not the same as medicalized embodiment, but instead are a supplemental register of sensation that is limited by sensory anatomy even as senses are excited over the edge of themselves'. We learn from Hayward that hormones change affective registers, thereby changing attentiveness and how embodied habits resonate. This (sometimes) fast tracks embodied change. Sensory shifts can support shifts in patterns of thought. Shifting embodied patterns can also stem from changing self-identification, but this requires a different attention.[84]

An example of a shift in thinking can be found in the process of attending the Gender Clinic. I (Mijke) was a performer and light technician, and while I had read a lot, my reading was not disciplined. The combined force of the two psychologists who were in control of the enforced process of diagnosis made me not only angry, because in moments of vulnerability I was met with violence and suspicion, but also showed me that I needed to train my thinking. I went on to study philosophy, to be able to counter these psychologists – in my words at that time, 'I want[ed] to build a bigger gun'. Thankfully, during my studies and especially after unlearning some of the patterns the philosophy department had demanded of me, I came to reject this image. I didn't want to have a proverbial gun; I wanted to change the pattern that made me want to think like a gun, a pattern that highlighted power over connection, that highlighted untouchability as good, rather than as a hindrance to flourishing. Because this was the power the psychologists wielded. The bellicose mode that I wanted to counter with another bellicose mode retained the formula of power and control. While being harassed and wounded by the psychologists at the clinic, it took a long time to question my complicity in maintaining such patterns. It took care, friends, reading, and conversations about dominance to understand where

I needed to shift. At the same time, my anarcho-communist background supported the embrace of those conclusions. I asked why in moments of stress these patterns come up, and how to change my mode of reacting, and ultimately my modes of sensing aggressions levied towards my way of being in the world. Did the hormones do that? No, but the awareness of shifting patterns of sensing – that was aided by my training as a dancer – and the awareness of how sensing, thinking, and responding are linked together, supported shifting modes of being in the world. Transness entails, in a way, finding new modes of attending to the world, with different sensitivities, and an openness to shifts in thinking. Transfeminism underlines these shifts to avoid atomist and categorical labels that emphasise stability, and perhaps simplicity, over change. Transfeminism questions how hierarchy slips into patterns of thought and action. We draw from various modes of thinking, and hold space for various modes of worlding – that is after all the fun of trans: it can be done in infinite ways that respond to each other. That is the basis for embracing the Zapatista slogan: *to have a world in which many worlds fit*, and to question how we need to change.

We close the chapter with a final thought on complicity. Lama Rod Owens's remark that *one can only hold people accountable for things they can change* might sound like a relief to some.[85] However, this statement can be understood to amplify one's responsibility for change. There is a *lot* we can change, both in ourselves and in collectives. And yet, there are structures that compel us to remain embedded in the world in harmful ways. Relying on indicating limits and oppressions can demobilise people, even if such a 'rigorous' analysis might seem to get to the heart of the matter. If there is no way to engage and do things differently, problems are sustained by introducing despair over organising our power. This is perhaps why highlighting totalising patterns is not part of our version of transfeminism. Instead of seeing hegemony as an inescapable system, we look at ways it is maintained and thereby find ways to break it down. Some of those ways have been learnt from Indigenous critiques on settler thinking, such as Mark Rifkin offers, some of those critiques have been learnt from Black liberation, such as Adrienne Maree Brown, and some of those have been learnt from European critics, such as Isabelle Stengers or Silvia Federici.[86] Embracing our own complicity maintains a sense of humility, which supports interdependence and underlines the need we have for each other's perspectives – the collectivity this generates is what is needed to counter the constraining aspects of our embodied life and how we can learn from others who live differently. There is no liberation without encountering our demons and facing them with different practices.

3

'It takes a nation of managers to hold us back'

Trans liberalism and liberation amid currents of empire

INTRODUCTION

In the UK, the backlash against trans and non-binary people has picked up on the wind of Brexit – the referendum that led to the UK's decision to leave the European Union, spurred on by far-right nationalist politicians, capital interests, and sentiments. Juxtaposed with the expansion and securitisation of the UK border into most aspects of public life, is the defence of a sex/gender binary reinscribed as essential to the maintenance of order, reinforced by the right-wing, including feminists, via legal bureaucracy, policing, and transphobic media. Attempts to defend the gender binary are by no means separated from the other assaults on civil liberties that the former Conservative Government undertook. Within this context, the government utilised the law to legitimise and 'streamline' bureaucracy to service the social exclusions and material divisions forged by racial capitalism and environmental destruction; to suppress dissent and the power forged by social movements and trade unions; and to hinder the agency of marginalised people by restricting access to rights, including reproductive rights. Key elements of these repressive legal tools are the widespread Hostile Environment policies and draconian approaches towards people seeking asylum;[1] additional powers given to police during and following the lockdowns for coronavirus and the upsurges in activity from Black Lives Matter since 2020 and Extinction Rebellion, manifest as the Policing, Crime, Sentencing and Courts Bill 2022, which suppresses the right to protest; and attempts to remove the jurisdiction of the European Court of Human Rights and to dismantle the UK's Human Rights Act 1998 and Equality Act 2010, through the proposed (although currently shelved) 'British Bill of Rights'.[2] Activists and non-governmental organisations continue to go to court to challenge the civil liberties and human rights that have been violated by such laws, while the government look for methods to short-circuit the power of the High and Supreme Courts.

In the liberal political sphere, calls for fairer representation and protection of rights are often proposed as tools to battle bias and social exclusion in the UK. It is within this framework that liberal trans activists, and non-governmental and third sector organisations, are pushing to pursue trans rights. Calls for trans rights tend to work as an open-ended political grammar – used by people and organisations with different political agendas – to broadly signify support for trans and non-binary people. But what specifically is denoted by 'trans rights' is varied and sometimes undefined. In the UK at the time of writing, the push for trans rights generally entails pursuing at least the following legal reforms:

A. Reforms to the Gender Recognition Act (2004), to make the legal recognition of trans people easier, including the removal of the need for medical certification of one's acquired gender, and to legally recognise the genders of non-binary people.[3] In Scotland, reforms have included allowing 16- and 17-year-olds to change their gender markers (within the gender binary), potentially making it easier to obtain other documents in one's chosen legal gender;[4]

B. Defence of the Equality Act (2010), which encodes the rights of trans and non-binary people, alongside other marginalised people, to be free from discrimination in the workplace, in hiring processes, and in accessing public services. In 2020, a landmark test case upheld the Equality Act to explicitly protect the rights of non-binary people;[5]

C. To challenge any proposals of 'bathroom bills' as seen in the US, or essentialist sex segregation in public services including hospitals, policed according to the legal marker on one's birth certificate, with fines threatened for those who transgress this;[6]

D. To fight for the legal right of trans youth to access gender-affirming healthcare, in the context of highly limited provisions;

E. To call upon governments to outlaw conversion therapies that target trans, non-binary and gender non-conforming people because of their gender non-conformity, which in the UK is in line with recent outlawing of conversion therapies targeting the sexualities of LGB people;

F. Pursuit of the right to be correctly gendered on the birth certificates of one's children, particularly in cases where trans men or trans-masculine people have given birth to a child.[7]

These are calls for the translation of the needs of trans and non-binary people into the framework of rights, bestowed by the state via law, proposing either reforms of bureaucracy and documentation to make them easier to navigate, or proposing that the right of access to public or state provisions and services for trans and non-binary people is ensured. There is an implicit assumption in the calls for trans rights that, in improving bureaucracy or affirming access to provisions, there will also be an improvement in the social and material conditions of trans and non-binary people. While this may seem logical, especially when it comes to accessing jobs and employment, it is not a given. This is especially critical given the kinds of material struggles and everyday discrimination that (especially poor and precarious) trans and non-binary people can face – in work, housing, education, healthcare and social life – even given the legal protections that we currently have.

In addition, the push for trans rights from more grassroots and left-leaning political organising includes:

G. To ensure that incarcerated trans people have access to gender-affirming materials, healthcare, legal gender recognition, while challenging discrimination in the housing of trans prisons and any proposals for 'trans prisons' from an abolitionist position;[8]

H. To increase, depathologise and/or fundamentally transform access and provisions for gender-affirming healthcare for all trans people (especially for those of us marginalised by the system due to racism, ageism and fatphobia), while creating collective and formal alternatives to the Gender Identity Clinic (GIC) system, including proposals to abolish these clinics and decentralise trans health care. These arguments emphasise that GICs remain rooted in socially conservative psychiatry in the UK (in spite of the official depathologisation of trans healthcare by WPATH), and that they function to limit the number of people who can access gender-affirming healthcare.[9]

While there is a clear need to access provisions such as work, housing and healthcare that are essential to survival in a capitalist society, approaches to improve lives through formal legal rights and through social solidarity and support are often collapsed into each other. This is consistent with a logic of identity politics which assumes that there are common social or political mutualities within the categories of trans and non-binary (e.g. that we are all left-leaning liberals, or that we are all 'woke'), and that the (unspecified) push for trans rights will thus benefit us all in the same manner. These are overarching logics of 'trans liberalism', which we will discuss below in detail in the context of the political climate of contemporary European nation-states. Such logics are contrasted by ethics and practices of *trans liberation* which entails solidarity and support to collectively transform our worlds. A more astute political grammar detangles the logics of trans liberalism from trans liberation, as part of a wider movement for social justice and total liberation. We will discuss how contemporary calls for trans rights, as delineated above, fall short of articulating a politics of liberation.

We write from the standpoint of activist scholars who have been embedded in various trans communities for the past two decades (primarily in the UK and the Netherlands), who are committed to solidarity across struggles and coalitional organising (including informally). We, and our colleagues and accomplices, have been active in collectives, groups, and formations that have put these more radical positions described above (points G and H) on the public agenda of current trans struggles. We understand trans liberation as bound up with the total liberation of all marginalised people, including survivors of abuse, incarcerated people, and all of us struggling for healthcare as disabled people, Mad people, and/or as racialised people and/or migrants living under racial capitalism with its ongoing colonial legacies. Liberation in this sense entails the dismantling of white supremacist, extractivist, ableist, cis- and heteronormative racial capitalism, and the power that this system and the nation-states that uphold it have over our ensouled bodyminds and lives, while also forming the conditions for the flourishing of life (we discuss this in Chapter 5). To speak a politics and language of liberation is to resonate with anti-colonial struggles against racial capitalism and empire, for the (collective) self-determination of Black, Brown, Indigenous and poor people, and marginalised groups (and, historically speaking, nations).[10] Trans and non-binary people living in colonial nations need to understand our relationship to the racial social infrastructures that cohere neoliberal nation-states, to which we are appealing for legal recognition. These are the infrastructures through which we all pass – some of us freely, while others of us face violence, incarceration or even death. We need to face how our 'demands' for trans rights as formal legal protections are *inextricable* from the legacies and ongoing forms of colonial dispossession and violence that the UK – or European – nation-states practice and represent. In the next section, we discuss how institutions function to individualise and restrict one's choices; and the need for collectives to shape their practices, such that they allow people to join in – even if, when compared to institutions, collectives fall apart more easily.

HUMAN RIGHTS FOR HUMAN RESOURCES:
INSTITUTIONAL STASIS AND INCLUSION

It is worth remembering that the international framework of Human Rights emerged in the mid-twentieth century, in a period where colonial nation-states worked to contain the influence and power of newly independent nations that had emerged through anti-colonial liberation movements.[11] Designated by nation-states and international bodies such as the UN, human rights were intended as the liberal and democratic protections of individuals or groups from states and exploitative corporations. In the present, a call for rights can function as either a demand to end an individual or group's exclusion from a state, and/or as the expression of an aspiration to be recognised as a full citizen.[12] Rights purport to offer a legal framework of protection, enabling opportunity and success, on terms that are governed by institutions and the state and are 'acceptable' to its dominant cultures. With rights, one is promised through inclusion the opportunity of enrichment in an *orderly* manner, whereby those who are marginalised (by social norms and pressures, by material conditions or geopolitical events and policies) are explicitly invited through law into the pre-existing legal and socio-economic structures of a nation. A legal emphasis – such as the bestowal of certain documents – might allow one to work when one was not permitted to before (such as being granted a work permit or Settled Status), but doesn't necessarily come with support from welfare or other material means.[13] In such a framework, problems, struggles and harms are considered in a nominal manner, and people are left to fend for themselves.

We are hesitant to rely on institutional and legal reforms for social change. Institutions curb our movements. Institutions function to stabilise the world, erecting fences to enable the control of an environment by management. Liberal institutions emerge from European Enlightenment philosophies ideas of knowledge and individual agency. In these theories, the boundaries of knowledge contain what can be controlled, while everything else is excluded as 'chaos'.[14] To be unknown is to have no place in the structure, which

entails not having access to the institutions that structure distri-
butions of attention and resources, and inform social hierarchy.[15]
Hence, a politics of inclusion functions to make one known within
the structure. The neoliberal reaction of the 1980s inaugurated a slow
transformation of society, proposing inclusion into the neoliberal
order through property, wealth, toeing the line of newly militarised
police states, while simultaneously dismantling and demobilising
labour – and in the 1990s, social – movements.[16] Neoliberalism
includes the infection of a 'morality-free' market logic into all strata
of life. This entails that both moral and political demands can only
be upheld if they appear to be financially responsible, and that both
public and private institutions too are brought under a regime of
financialisation. Social life is, famously in the words of Margaret
Thatcher, reduced to individuals and families, each of which must
effectively become 'entrepreneurs of their own life', while the welfare
state is dismantled. Hence, social movements with more complex
and far-ranging demands that aim to re-organise social space are
both blocked by a manufactured 'realism' of finance and policy, and
cast out beyond the fences of society, labelled – as in the case of
the anti-racist movements of the 1980s – as chaotic swarms. Four
decades on, the extent to which inclusion in institutions produces
stasis and relies on demobilising social movements is evident.

As Moten proposes, the political space of citizenship and
participation in institutions is the space of anti-sociality and coun-
ter-relationality.[17] Sociality is submerged under the perfecting
demands of production. Standards of perfection and purification
structure the public and institutional realm of the citizen by stripping away blossoming varieties of life. Institutions are not just
regulated to close out outsiders, they are the barriers against unruly
relationalities that are not subject to the forces that constitute the
citizens inside(s). Fortress Europe, and its escalation Brexit Britain,
are not new political interventions, because closure is the foundation of European hegemony. This closure is partly structured by
epistemologies that cannot acknowledge an outside to the institutional frame.

Meanwhile, individualism is encouraged through a language of individual wishes and wants; individualisation is a necessary element of the process of inclusion. The emphasis on the individual safeguards institutions against collectivised pressure. Included individuals, especially of marginalised groups, are easily isolated and controlled amid the dominant currents of the institution; the wider social pressures that lead to marginalisation can be addressed superficially in the institutional context. Organisational structures that emphasise managerial control are shaped in such a way that allows space for individual decisions – this even, sometimes, goes by the name of autonomy (as we discuss regarding healthcare in the next chapter). Yet the range of choices is limited in possibility and scope by organisational hierarchies. 'Freedom of choice' offers only pre-determined options already shaped by institutions, even if in the moment of making a choice it is experienced as going against the grain. This modicum of individual agency is key to the dissolution of collective agency and collaboration in social movements. Conversely, movements can remake social forms without hierarchy, through collective vision and action. When we exercise our agency against institutions as individuals, we often end up burnt out.

While this picture might seem bleak, it offers a chance to rethink freedom of choice and its attendant term autonomy. Collective liberation asks much more of us – in terms of responsibility, action, and a preparedness to relinquish personal wishes. In Chapter 1, we discussed the femme work of making groups into collectives, which includes the way they come together and act (perhaps) in concert. When we think of liberation with regard to collectives, we provoke ourselves into stepping out of hierarchies, including the fragmentation and enforced separation that racial capitalism produces, while refusing the logics of accumulation and separability.[18] Collectives function differently than institutions, because the possibility of refusal of participation infuses a non-hierarchical element. A call to action might be met with inertness, people might stop showing up, or simply ignore what is said. This is not always bad, for instance, it might mean that a group is not ready to deal with a situation, or it might mean that certain methods of social organisation are not acceptable, or people disagree on an outcome. In this way movement work contrasts managerial hierarchies that purport to 'get things done'.

In collectives when people do not show up, one is aware that things are not going well. In contrast, when in institutions people do not show up, it means that they are not generating friction within its functioning, which is taken as indication that all is going well. Collectives come together in many ways, which need to be learnt or rehearsed, to create shared outcomes. Yet, collectives do not provide pre-determined choices for existing questions, because part of the collective work is to shape the future one wants to live.[19] Choice is substituted by the necessity to create futures in the present, which involves shaping practices in a manner that supports engagement of the collective's members. However, it is also a common occurrence that collectives fall apart. Such falling out can be painful for the people involved, although it can also be understood as inevitable for the distribution of knowledge. Fallouts make possible the transfer of knowledge and methods to new groups, the combining of knowledges from different organisations. Although, in comparison to institutions, such fallouts can appear to be a sign of the unfeasibility of horizontal organising, rather than a sign of its success. Collectives are partly about making new relations, because by coming together imaginations are formed, knowledge is transferred, and forms of being together are explored and developed. Creating a present in which futures can be conceived does not work in every group that comes together, which is not necessarily a bad thing. We offer this here to provide a foothold to the contrast between institutions and collectives. In the concluding chapter, we develop a collective ethics more deeply. The analysis sketched above frames how we see trans liberation and freedom from oppression.

Institutions operate on the postulate of a seemingly coherent structure with various interlocking levels, maintaining its function amid daily changes, small ruptures, and challenges. Institutional power is formed of distributed agency on various levels that function within a hierarchy of control. Such power is both overwhelming and nuanced: overwhelming, because it reaches various levels by means of its distribution; and nuanced, because it individualises its members and participants, and gives them choices in how to respond, even to (dis)align with the institution. For instance, through the ostentatious claim to privacy or freedom of speech, one is free to have any opinion in one's 'own' time, while embedded in the structure during 'work' time.[20] This dual motion of privatised morality and public order through law, policy, and norms lays claim to freedom as well as stability.[21]

The political right especially claims to be defenders of freedom, constructed primarily through freedom of speech without accountability. Amidst the racist, xenophobic and anti-trans backlash, a notable exception is freedom of choice for women. Sayak Valencia writes:

> In my opinion, the prohibition of abortion in the state is a distraction tactic of patriarchal institutions, represented by doctors, fathers, priests, lovers, rapists, etc., so as not to have to speak of themselves or about the ultraviolent context in which Baja California lives on a daily basis. Talking constantly about women, their bodies, their sexuality, and their choices is the best way to continue controlling us; it's a clear way to avoid the enunciation of an autonomous discourse about their own issues. As Virginie Despentes states: 'Men like to talk about women. That way, they don't have to talk about themselves.'[22]

Liberals respond to this ideological onslaught by defending freedom as freedom of choice. Liberal freedom of choice means choosing between pre-figured options, as we have argued above, which can be claimed as one's own – a hallmark of a possessive individualism.[23] Liberty in this form means to exercise agency in a splendid isolation. Such isolation makes one necessarily collapse back into the norm, even if one wishes to escape from duress, or simply live a life less ordinary. Individualised agency can only get one so far, even though in the hubristic Eurocentric imagination an individual has the power to change the world. As imperialism shows, changing the world requires a system, a form of power that allows for the intentions of a few to be channelled through an institutional framework supported by laws and policies.[24] This kind of institutionalisation is a mode of world-making.[25] This form of world-making comes with an action-orientation and self-understanding aptly called *subjectivity:* one is subject in and to the systems one understands oneself within – a little ruler in a little realm. María Lugones calls individualised agency the domain of 'managers, foremen, lesser officials, and upholders of the institutional apparatus'.[26] According to Lugones, individualised power can only be exercised when backed by institutions. This power is also curbed to what is *possible* within institutional logics – if individual power means to 'successfully' manifest intentions in the world, it is severely limited in the scope of which intentions *can be* manifested. The idea of individual power, therefore, buttresses current structures and energy spent can at best create variations on pre-determined themes. And yet, despite this analysis, claiming personal choices seems inevitable for the demand – our demand – that we have autonomy over our bodies: our bodies, our choice.

To delve further into this, in universities an emphasis on individual agency and managerial power interlock to create freedom of content and simultaneously reinforce hierarchy. In the 1990s, the increasing precarity of contracts coincided with an emboldening of hierarchy in academic workplaces (often in the name of market logics and executive pay). The enforcement of managerial command of the structure of the institution at the same time allowed individual lecturers to shape courses according to their own ethical commitments. Crucially, we can see that it is *because* of inclusion and precarity, that control of course content is devolved to individual lecturers. Especially precarious engagements come with a freedom in regard to the syllabus, because the control that is rescinded on course content (a retraction of moralising homogeneity) is subsumed by a control over structures (an emphasis on financial authority), which often relies on quantified data on spreadsheets. This novel patriarchy is not commandeering, but managerial.[27] The stasis of relations dries up the impetus for social change.[28] However, an often-derided managerial lack of vision, in conjunction with meaningless marketing slogans, also undergirds the possibility of working against the 'erasure' of certain topics.[29]

However, the inclusion of marginalised knowledges demands abandonment of organisational forms that are integrated with counter-normative approaches. It remains an open question whether such inclusion in fact works against erasure or co-opts and neutralises knowledges to become institutionally accessible.[30] Such adaptations might merely give an illusion that all kinds of knowing fit in a single patriarchal organisational form. And still, the institutional structure might include previously ignored perspectives, even if these outsider knowledges might be captured by controlling normativities. For instance, top-down policy requires data to be sent upwards via schemes of evaluation, which might determine hiring policies. Schemes of evaluation adapt insights into institutional structures. Metrics function to keep control of the output, irrespective of content – in this sense institutions can grant freedom while retaining control. Depersonalising the means of evaluation, through policy and metrics, disguises patriarchal disinterest with a sheen of objectivity: the interest of the institution is in representation (of results, metrics, diversity, ranking, grants, outputs), but not in connection. The managerial middle literally guards the norm and demands adaptation and alignment by issuing reports, harvesting data from classroom and research activity, controlling processes, and strutting up organisations against the influence of staff. Inclusion comes at the price of disempowerment. Disempowerment is necessary, because knowledge (about duress, social pressure, economic marginalisation) that needs to be considered hinders the top-down operation of power. Marginalisation is thus a foundational prerequisite of institutions *because* of the refusal to be accountable.

A call for trans rights aims to open doors and remove obstacles. But, as we argued above, incorporation into a managerial structure in institutions can hinder transformation, as collective movements are reduced to individual positions. Put simply, to occupy an institutional position as trans 'activist' might mean that one's personal conditions are improved, and one's individual voice is amplified – yet, the level of empowerment that one gains on the individual level might come to block gains in collective power. Individual empowerment (whether through fame, institutional position, social hierarchy, etc.) can disrupt the careful creation of social relations that require *distributed* agency.[31] Institutions rely on alignment with their structures, to the point that one has to see oneself as personally responsible for maintaining institutions in the form of deep adherence to policy or law, as argued by Kantian philosophers. Not doing so, in these philosophies, is evil.[32] Navigating institutional incorporation by oscillation between (seeming) alignment and refusal of institutional patterns is key to surviving inclusion. Refusal of institutional norms leads to a refusal of institutional oversight, and this refusal can be structured around the commitment to abolition.

SEPARABILITY AND THE LAW OF GENDER

Bureaucracy functions to maintain order, to lubricate the status quo and to establish on paper who is part of the order, and who is kept out of it.[33] As shown by the recent endeavours to improve the situation of legal gender recognition for trans people and, to varying degrees, for non-binary people, alongside questions that regularly appear in equal opportunities monitoring,[34] law and neoliberal governance continue to consider the legal role of gender or 'sexgender' as of central importance to their functioning. Given that there is no legal distinction between sex and gender in the UK, critical feminist legal scholars use 'sexgender' to denote this concept as it functions in law. The current Gender Recognition Act in the UK permits the legal change of one's sex within the gender binary (male/female), provided that one's chosen gender is signed off by a doctor, and that one meets the criteria of demonstrating one's gender change set and judged by a bureaucratic panel. The very possibility of legal gender recognition is better than none. However, the difficulty in negotiating this bureaucratic process, the outmoded gender norms that have been upheld by the Gender Identity Clinics (with little leeway until very recently), the cost of making this application prior to its reduction in 2021, and the limited bureaucratic use of birth certificates themselves, have all functioned to deter potential applicants.

Indeed, only 5,871 GRCs were issued between its introduction in 2005 and late 2020.[35] All of these limiting aspects – and especially the limits of the legal gender binary itself, demonstrate the state's regulation and control of trans legal status.

Grietje Baars considers how law upholds gender, 'what work the *legal* category of gender does in (re)producing the cisheteropatriarchy', and that 'gender is one of the last remaining state-assigned and supposedly stable and permanent "characteristics" of a person that remains explicitly registered as a key element of one's *legal* "identity" in most countries around the world'.[36] Gender (sexgender) *as a legal category* has upheld cisgenderism – which is, as theorised by Gavriel Ansara, an ideology that works through distinctions (F and M) 'to delegitimise people's self-designations', of our 'genders and bodies by external actors'[37] – to maintain order in the nation-state. Cisgenderism is 'a form of "othering" that takes people categorised as "transgender" as "the effect to be explained"' – it is *systemic* and multi-layered. The practices of delegitimisation that uphold cisgenderism occur 'during everyday interactions with societal systems'.[38] It may also involve practices of de-gendering in everyday speech where trans people are described in gender-neutral terms, over and beyond when this is our preference, or with the use of essentialist or 'objectifying biological language'.[39]

Legal reform regarding gender recognition proposes to fix the cisgenderist function of legal gender, through allowing for self-identification of one's gender, for instance. However, self-identification does not question the role of legal gender itself, as is considered in recent scholarship on gender decertification.[40] Non-binary inclusion through the adoption of an X option proposes to add a third legal gender to the binary categories. As legal genders continue to be assigned at birth,[41] both to the child and in most cases to their parents too, there remains an onus on the individual to raise an issue with their state-assigned gender, to lodge one's status as different and provide an explanation, through whatever administrative protocol – often invasive and/or medicalising – that is required to change it. Furthermore, the legal function of gender can raise challenges for non-binary and trans parents, such as trans men and non-binary people who give birth.

Baars discusses multiple 'Queer Cases' regarding trans and non-binary people in examples from Germany, Israel, and the UK, where trans men who give birth are legally defined as 'mothers', over-riding their legal status as male, because legal systems remain wedded to an essentialist, heteronormative and of course cis-normative understanding of sexual reproduction.[42] For Baars, the 'Straight Court' seems to lack a critical capacity to register in law either the possibilities or realities of trans sexual reproduction. Despite the logical possibility of simply registering 'parents' in a non-gendered fashion, or of couples who have had gay marriages being legal parents to a child, Baars underlines that courts uphold the idea that children are born of cisgender people, where the rights of a child are invoked to trump those of a trans parent. The systematic imposition of legal gender has lasting effects from gendered assignments at birth, with additional complications for people who are intersex and/or those of us who transition and change legal gender. Legal gender seems essential to the state's distribution of power, and contesting its categorisations can influence one's status as a citizen, one's material opportunities, and degrees of discrimination. Gender decertification is proposed as one tool in 'dismantling a legal structure that institutionalises gender-based categories' – categories that are socially unequal – undermining the naturalisation of gender divisions, and removing the burden of legal cisgenderism on trans and non-binary people.[43]

Amid limited and sometimes precarious forms of legal and social inclusion, the role of bureaucracy to maintain order has become pronounced, as nation-states and institutions find themselves trying to defend their (apparently diminishing) resources for the purposes of their dominant subjects and capital interests. Inclusion for some is promised by the left hand, while the exclusion of others is rekindled by the right, all within a context of further checks and controls. As we discuss below, the UK state continues to reproduce dynamics of empire through legal and policing endeavours, including within its mainland borders. This includes, since the mid-2010s, the entrenchment of the UK border into many crucial aspects of public life through the Hostile Environment policy. This policy limits access to essential resources and services (housing, health-care, welfare, employment, education, and the right to reside in the UK), which in turn adversely affects Black, Brown, migrant people, including trans people, disproportionately, and creates bureaucratic problems for some trans people with UK passports. This policy is a key aspect of the architecture of a state committed to the further bureaucratisation and surveillance of public life, which is fed by xenophobic and anti-Black ideology[44] in the pursuit and produc-tion of strategies of separability.

Separability, proposed by Denise Ferreira da Silva, is a key concept to understand the creation and maintenance of social hier-archies.[45] Separability describes dividing the population into those who are welcome to the table, those who own the building and order the streets surrounding it; and those who are exploited to give the meeting legitimacy, to harvest produce that is served up or to clean up afterwards, or are left out for disposal or death. Separability is essential to the functioning of racial capitalism, as it stabilises its social hierarchies and divisions of labour, access, and wealth. Da Silva discusses how bureaucratisation in service of the border is a current trend for the defence of Fortress Europe from those who are racialised, migrants or refugees, who are understood to be different and therefore legitimately excluded.[46] The abstract idea of 'others' leads to additional policing of Black and Brown people – often stig-matised by Islamophobic sentiments – fleeing conflicts, seeking safety, and/or opportunity, 29,325 of whom have lost their lives in trying to reach Europe since 2014.[47] At this moment of economic, health and climate crises, the hoarding and 'protection' of resources and of land, and growing investment in the economies of military and defence by corporations and wealthy nation-states is deemed essential in the attempt to expand capitalist accumulation – at the continued expense of human life and planetary ecologies. The coro-navirus pandemic revealed a key truth of racial capitalism once again: that lives, especially those of people who are already marginalised by race, class, ability, and age, are disposable to the ruling classes (even if it leads to a devastating labour shortage).

In considering the Hostile Environment as a strategy of separability – as we discuss this later in the chapter – we can read how governments and centre and right-wing media stoke divisions as a 'culture war', which in turn can have serious material effects. State and media-endorsed transphobia and racism ('war on woke') are both drivers of separation and divisive affective economies – functioning respectively to turn trans women, non-binary people and trans people more broadly into scapegoats of cultural decadence gone too far, who are undermining an (essentialist) gender binary; and to delegitimise the political analysis of intellectuals, activists and cultural workers challenging racism and Britain's colonial legacies, especially that of Black and Brown women and femmes. These forms of hatred deploy *generalising* stereotypes – of trans women or trans people in accordance with a limited cissexist imaginary of what we look like, of what our bodies are,[48] or of woke intellectuals teaching critical race theory to minors or adults. These denunciations of trans people or anti-racist intellectuals occur through targeted media assassinations and social media harassment, complete with slurs and death threats. Transphobic feminists attempt to uphold an essentialist gender binary that aligns with the nation-state as empire and its conservative institutional powers, which in turn use bureaucracy to segregate access to essential resources along the lines of citizenship, race, and religion.

Moments of obnoxious violence enacted by conservatives (including transphobic feminists) hide an anxiety and fear of the social change and transformation ushered in by trans and non-binary people, as we eclipse the worldview wedded to empire and the gender binary. These fears are related to the xenophobic fears of 'migrants coming over here and taking our jobs' – fears that themselves are founded in either an erasure of coloniality and a lack of understanding of global labour markets, or the valorisation of coloniality, its expropriation of resources and an unequal global racial and gendered division of labour.[49] Obnoxious attitudes draw on the entitlement of white supremacy and the valorisation of coloniality (e.g. claiming that Britain civilised the people it colonised and that this was an unquestioned good), and together with fear and its related affects, organise to guard the norm against transgression, transformation, and destabilisation. Together, fear, obnoxiousness, and the hatred of difference promote a sense of scarcity, encouraging allocating resources and space only to those who are privileged by norms, but who claim this as their 'right'. The ongoing transfer of wealth upwards, towards the super-rich and the ruling capitalist classes, remains out of focus of these claims – and we increasingly see claims of victimisation being made from within these classes. The resources and spaces in question are moreover already spoils of empire and exploitation. All the while, those conforming to the norm lack the breadth of awareness that they're *already* sharing spaces with marginalised people, unable to see this unless marginalisation is 'visible'.

This mix of fear of 'others', hatred of difference, obnoxiousness, entitlement, and anxieties regarding social change, are channelled into the development of bureaucratic governance and policing of access to resources. Bureaucracy functions to exclude those less able to navigate administrative spaces (through obstacles that may include language, ableism, correct documents, or other things), while those who know how to navigate them can access resources. Those who move in the flow of norms of whiteness, citizenship, migration status, sexuality, and gender are able to access resources, even with the introduction of increased surveillance and identity checks (passport checks) throughout daily life. The Hostile Environment works to affront Black and Brown people – reducing and preventing access to resources by targeting asylum seekers, refugees or people without recourse to public funds in particular, alongside people with precarious immigration status. Bureaucratisation engenders distress, harm, and even violence to those of us who are marginalised, face questioning, and may have our integrity thrown into doubt; this dovetails with prejudices platformed by the conservative and liberal media and politicians. While having documents does make a difference, the threat of administrative violence has been dramatically increased and spread out through society with the Hostile Environment. Anyone who, on a given day, doesn't pass in the norm, may be stopped at the border, a border now dispersed into everyday life. The border in the everyday is not upheld consistently: with the legislative changes that made certain workers within public office responsible for undertaking document checks for the Home Office, some individuals responsible for these checks may be lenient, actively ignoring the Prevent duty[50] or working against restrictions. Others may throw the full force of their position into the operation of the bureaucracy, perhaps to compensate for perceived lenience by others. Such border checks and the degrees of uncertainty further heighten anxieties, feeding into division and separability.

Trans struggles in Brexit Britain, Fortress Europe, and the wider landscape of far-right powers, need to address how inclusion into the institutions of neoliberal capitalist society and nation-states through rights will produce markedly more benefit for some over others, and doesn't address the complex material conditions currently facing people – through race and class, immigration status, religion, ability, and gender. Enfranchisement through rights does not directly correlate to an improvement of material or economic conditions for marginalised people, especially if we are facing extreme forms of bureaucracy, policing, and surveillance, and serious economic hardship. Trans and non-binary folks who are considered to be respectable and acceptable to the social norm may be welcomed (back) into its fold, with the *promise* of comfort and belonging. However, conceiving of the enfranchisement of trans people as the enfranchisement of a homogeneous minority group via law is *not* a politic of liberation. It is demonstrative of a politic that is sliding into further entanglement with a neocolonial state through inclusion within it. Liberal trans politics has so far failed to meaningfully challenge the widespread violence of the Hostile Environment and the reinforcement of borders throughout everyday Brexit Britain. Trans rights do not immediately tend to the liberation of trans and non-binary people, and other urgent material issues are not being addressed in the *discourses* around rights. As Mijke writes, 'Rights might protect one from management, but they will not liberate one from it'.[51]

Indeed, a transfeminist ethics, the practice of care and solidarity, are ways to manifest alternatives of support, survival, and nourishing worlds, while challenging and dismantling the separability of white supremacist states and cultural logics. Through this ethics, we practice the refusal of a system that enacts dispossession and harm, that mobilises separability as a contemporary form of segregation. The ethics of care and solidarity described in the book can bring relief from the extremity of material struggles, helping to establish a ground from which liberation can emerge. Next, we unpack the politics of trans liberalism, and consider the capture of practices of liberation in the contemporary political and economic climate.

TRANS LIBERALISM AMID CURRENTS OF EMPIRE AND NEOFASCISM

'Trans liberalism' describes a political logic that pursues equality through legal rights and recognition, foregrounding the importance of inclusion into social, economic, legal, and cultural institutions. This politics claims 'transgender rights are *the solution* to the problems facing trans people'; that trans rights 'will enable our participation in (Western) capitalist society; that, alongside rights, positive media representation is the best method to win over the cisgender world and [to] improve the standing of trans subjects within the multicultural diversity of an apparently equal society'.[52] By promoting overtly positive trans visibility, alongside sometimes highlighting aspects of our struggles, as a cultural politics it endeavours to improve public attitudes towards trans and non-binary people.[53] Inclusion through rights endeavours to correct biases within pre-existing legal and social systems (that is, bureaucratic systems that assume cisnormativity as discussed above), such that trans (and potentially non-binary) people may be accepted within these systems. Trans liberalism is a form of neoliberal multiculturalism, a politic that promotes the attitudes of tolerance, diversity and equality under capitalism.[54] Such multiculturalism has been mobilised by political leaders and NGOs since the 1990s – and while out-of-fashion at the time of writing, has been promoted by the likes of Tony Blair, Angela Merkel, and Nicola Sturgeon. This cultural politics correctly understands that negative representations lead to discrimination; however, it fails to understand that exclusion is a necessary outcome of the social organisation of a capitalist society, and that such exclusions are the result of social hierarchies which have emerged historically with the functioning of racial capitalism, necessary for the extraction of resources and labour. Trans liberalism proposes to reform legal, social and cultural institutions to make them more inclusive, rather than bringing the structure of institutions into question and asking whether abolishing institutions might better serve the lives of marginalised people.

In coming out as trans or non-binary, one may find oneself shocked at being excluded from social systems, a shock that challenges one's assumptions about this world, one's access to social and legal institutions and the possibilities that they engender, alongside shifts in access to public space. These assumptions are often built upon whiteness, being able-bodied, heteronormativity, and increasingly homonormativity. Accommodations for trans and non-binary people have taken the form of adjustments such as providing gender-neutral bathrooms, the use of correct pronouns, and sometimes the administrative recognition of gender on the terms described by trans and non-binary people [M/F/X], and provisions of (sometimes gender-specific) services to trans and non-binary people in a sensitive manner. We name these aspects in particular, as they are the primary issues that we've seen raised over the last ten to fifteen or so years, including the period around the 'transgender tipping point' in 2014.[55] These outcomes and institutional policies have emerged from practices in self-organised trans and queer communities – those of us from these communities actively raising what are fairly basic needs. The resulting changes are not transformational of the structures that they are made within. Bathrooms in universities, offices and cultural centres may become gender-neutral; stating one's pronouns alongside one's name and using they/them to address someone in the gender-neutral third person is becoming increasingly commonplace in institutional spaces. However, other structural dynamics do not get addressed by such changes – such as the grip and power of a highly salaried managerial class, when workers have faced serious real-term pay cuts since the mid-2000s.

While the politics of trans liberalism – in the context of an anti-trans backlash – receives support from non-governmental organisations and charities, committees, or particular government departments, and grassroots activists and individuals, it does not deliver an analysis of the structural effects of inclusion. It seems that inclusion is an end in itself. Indeed, LGBTQI+ issues have sometimes been framed as 'merely cultural' or social issues, as questions of diversity and 'minority' rights, by commenters and theorists across the political spectrum. This is far from the case – as studies and journalistic accounts on the experiences of LGBTQ people of, for instance, mental distress, workplace harassment, and homelessness have repeatedly shown that trans people are overrepresented in facing negative experiences, pointing to the material issues that underlie problems we are more likely to face.[56] The material conditions facing trans and non-binary people from *structural* transphobia remain a problem. One may still experience interpersonal discrimination that affects access to work, education, housing, or healthcare, the impacts of which can have serious lasting effects on one's life, living conditions and/or health. A concrete example is that despite discrimination at work or in the hiring process based on gender or gender identity being outlawed by the Equality Act 2010, a 2021 Totaljobs survey found that 33% of trans people had experienced discrimination in applying and interviewing for jobs, and 32% reported having 'experienced discrimination or abuse at work in the last five years'.[57]

Inclusion assumes that legal enfranchisement will drive an improvement in social and cultural *attitudes* towards marginalised people – an assumption that there are 'trickle-down' effects from rights. It is also assumed that legal enfranchisement will necessarily improve the *material conditions* of marginalised groups. Inclusion assumes that, for trans people, having incorrect documents is the primary challenge when accessing work or education or housing or healthcare. While the ability to change one's name and gender marker on a passport or driving licence (which, while expensive and stressful, is possible to do within the F/M gender binary) makes accessing work or education or housing or healthcare a little easier, non-binary people are left with the problem of having to out themselves within these contexts.

Neil Stammers argues that in the move from activists 'demanding' rights to institutions implementing rights, a shift in meaning happens. Stammers proposes that social movements have an expressive dimension – that is beyond identity – and also an instrumental dimension: that a movement fights for concrete political, economic, and social demands and 'that such demands do not necessarily serve the interests of [only] those actors'.[58] The expressive side of social movements focuses on 'values, norms, lifestyles, identities, symbols, discourses, etc.'[59] For Stammers, this tension is a general dialectic of social movements, which varies in its particulars between movements and across time and space. The demand for rights is intended as a challenge to power, and the expressive side of a movement establishes a 'counter-hegemonic' understanding of the issue at the level of the public – it makes power visible, and makes those disempowered visible in a new light. Our critique lies in the focus on the possibility of rights. While a demand for rights might initially work to challenge power, the move to consolidate some of the gains sustains power by handing over protection to a centralised institution, and thus impedes further change. What emerges is that rights are spurring cultural change, while at the same time hindering transformative change, by limiting movements according to institutional realism.

Trans movements seem to go through cycles of mobilisation and demobilisation – a pattern that Stammers lays out as recognisable in contemporary movements more broadly – in part by failing to retain recent historical memory. Protest is *ad hoc* and supported by negotiations of NGOs that are (at times) the result of the expressive side of movements, although are not best suited to challenge structural issues of distribution. A downside of liberal movements is exactly this limitation to a politics of representation, which primarily concerns identity, and (perceived) interests expressed through rights. The 2010s saw a shift from a social-economic analysis to a cultural analysis in trans politics, which meant that trans politics became depoliticised and rarely focused on solidarity.[60] The current framing of trans movements around rights – and focus on GRA reform, legal recognition and autonomy (in healthcare settings) in the UK – are at best a ticket into a job market where the rest of the structural nightmare and discriminations of racial, ableist capitalism will still meet us; where we *may* be freer to travel and access what is otherwise fenced off for us by the state. A transfeminist ethics by contrast aims to feed and cultivate possibilities and dreams, how we make our lives together, while ending everyday duress and traumatic harms. Legal reforms at this moment – the achievement of which already feels far-fetched in many places, unless some more supposedly compassionate managers enter government – will not address the pressing issues of our times.

However, it is important to acknowledge that, in parallel, individual empowerment of members of formerly excluded social groups within institutions leads to people putting effort into support and mentorship. In the face of challenges to split our political movements – by active stances against non-binary and trans participation in grassroots and party politics, or in attempts by neoliberal states to co-opt and defang our movements, claiming credit for successes of trans communities and activists, while pinkwashing and rainbow capitalism sells rainbow flags back to us – we need to address the stakes that we share, and discuss the concrete particulars of our struggles across imposed divisions. As Che Gossett has remarked, it is not particularly liberating to be arrested by a trans cop.[61] Similarly, as when we will discuss medical care in the next chapter, we need to be careful when relying on individual empowerment as a spearpoint for thinking through institutional change and its relationship with autonomy (as individual choice), that is 'demanded'. The language of demand in rights discourses is interesting in the sense that it keeps hierarchies in place: one asks those in power to bestow a right and in that sense maintains the existing relations of power. We are wary of a trans politics that can only use the same language as management: the *demand* for 'trans rights now' suggests that our political grammar has stalled.

KNOW YOUR TRANS RIGHTS NOW

With a constricted perspective, liberal trans politics focuses on removing social obstacles and challenging institutional exclusion. Such a politics relies on the individual experience of limitations. This framework emerges from an Enlightenment ideology that duress stems from a lack of understanding that needs to be addressed, and it is assumed that a better understanding will lead to a greater acceptance of trans people. In practice, the emphasis on knowledge and limitation leads to a focus on speaking from one's direct experience as an experience of 'pain and hurt' to emphasise structural limitations to inclusion. A similar pattern can be seen as with institutional inclusion: replacing a 'movement consciousness' with experience gives everyone a claim to be a knowledge producer at the price of individualising struggles: I am asked to speak about my experiences of limitations, while that form of speaking is taken to be constitutive of my 'identity'. These narratives are taken to be stand-ins for understanding social structures. Personal experiences of obstructions are taken to be representative of general oppression, rather than as a mapping of localised perspectives.[62] For example, my struggles within a university are indeed related to me being trans – yet, the narrative takes for granted that I'm in a university, which also means that I (likely) have a residency permit, some form of income that allows me to be there, a certain access to language, understanding of bureaucracy, and class-based interactions. Most likely my healthcare is covered, and I might have food.

While we might say that it takes friction to become aware of one's limitations, we might also say that it takes curiosity, care, and political consciousness. A middle-class worldview, or academic worldview, limits itself often to a struggle over 'who is right' – rather than take contrasting views, or proposals for actions as simply different proposals, between which you can choose because the choice is not based on a hierarchy of insight (where some views being 'better'). Middle-classness, especially a Eurocentric one, demands a single, shared worldview, where deviations are cast as limitations, stunted development (as in misogyny, trans and queerphobia) or dehumanising difference (in racialisation). When obstructions to knowledge are seen as the problem, a logical political strategy is to focus on avoiding misrepresentation.

Struggle for inclusion has at its heart a politics of representation. Such a fight for inclusion bases a politics on identity, rather than an identity on politics.[63] Identity comes to rest 'upon an assumptive coherence, knowability, and nonporousness, all of which are regulated, normative regimes of legibility and stability'.[64] A politics of representation overlooks the severity of duress at the margins, while offering a worldview that relies on the homogenisation of identity.[65] Trans representation that focuses on providing better understanding to majorities can avoid addressing one's responsibilities within harmful structures. Meanwhile, majoritarian 'innocence' is affirmed by admitting to a lack of knowledge, and trans issues are presented by trans actors with access to institutions. Activism from such a worldview places megaphones in the hands of those who wield narratives and politics in a way that structurally empowered people can find reasonable. This results in a two-way alignment: the struggle against exclusion comes from an acceptable perspective, and those in power can choose to give attention to those who they find comprehensible, rather than having to change their own worldview. While a politics of inclusion invites structural change to end exclusion of an 'identity', identity remains a categorical reference to those (formerly) excluded, shoring up normative thinking in categories, stabilising patterns of difference and separability.[66]

Once included, minoritised actors need to fend for themselves, while ensuring they fit into structures that might or might not promote their flourishing. In contrast, an identity based on politics bases its premise on the inverse: the direction of struggle is what forms one's affiliation. Marquis Bey writes, 'Being put in a box says little about how one occupies that box and how others relate to that box'.[67] To speak relevantly about trans liberation struggles, means that I need to transcend the limitations of my perspective and extend outside of my experience. My experience of limitations does not encompass the entire category of trans, indeed it might miss significant portions of it. Experience does not limit the scope of one's politics, but invites dealing with one's limitations, received duress, frictions, and perspective. Solidarity work relies on opening up sensitivities, building knowledge, skills, and curiosity to do things differently, which includes the willingness to give up one's habits, question one's perspectives, and hold different and contrasting views as complementary, rather than contradictory. Our argument for complicity returns at this stage as a way to map one's participation in an environment and see how this shrinks or expands one's understanding of actions, methods and socialities. To embrace complicity means to question which commitments might undergird one's position, and consequently, what an ethics of solidarity might look like. This kind of politics does not rest with inclusion but attends to wider solidarities.

Thinking in identities seems to be complicated by trans lives that lean on statements of the fluidity of being, sometimes as a claim against normative legibility. These claims may range from being grounded in disruptive and transformative practices, to a self-understanding that refrains from unsettling one's social (or material) position. We could say that social change is slow, and the weight of the norm is hard to escape; yet we could also acknowledge that a stronger focus on building alternative forms of life is perhaps where foundational fluidity or difference is found. When one tracks trans lives through the decennia by means of activist groups, like Street Transvestite Action Revolutionaries (STAR), Gay Liberation Front in the UK, and various groups aimed at liberation from capitalist pressures in a colonial world, we can see that gendered fluidity was a part of that liberation work, but never a stand-alone issue.

Currently, gender fluidity seems to have lost this foundational momentum towards broader solidarity. We got out of the box, but immediately got stuck. This seems to be the result, in part, of casting fluidity or indeterminacy as counteridentification to dominant normative categorisations, rather than emerging from a broader political-epistemic aim.[68] This shows in moments when a plurality of perspectives emerges, that dismissing the dominant manner of speaking (or the ghost of assumptions about hegemony) becomes the refrain, while there is a considerable lack of experience in how to practically work with differences in a manner that is not alienating. Muñoz's understanding of *disidentification* can reinvigorate exploring of forms of life. Disidentification is proposed as a movement that tactically misrecognises norms as a form of active resistance rather than a reactive retort to normative pressures. Especially, in this moment where trans people are made to respond to their 'interests' in the form of legal recognition, sanitary access, and institutional accommodation, actively shaping alternatives can reinvigorate trans politics. The idea of gender fluidity did not liberate, but rather started to function as a boundary not to question why our lives did not remarkably change, despite years of activist work.[69] The avoidance of a radical ethics by focusing on identity hinders movement building and thereby actual liberation.

The lesser focus on building movement skills also creates moments where people, who are hoping to have their feelings or experiences validated, feel that in activist circles they (again) need to take a step back. Without skills and methods that make this palatable, fragmentation is bound to happen. As we wrote in Chapter 2, care is one mode of attending to people's needs in movements, another is to work towards forms of organising that keep engagements open and do not enforce hierarchies. An embrace of solidarity without homogeneity can make possible difference without leading to separability too. Da Silva explains, '[w]ithout *separability*, difference among human groups and between human and non-human entities, has very limited explanatory purchase and ethical significance'.[70] A politics of solidarity situates our differences in connection, where working towards liberation is a shared endeavour. A politics of demands, aimed at institutions, fragments collective needs by forcing them to be presented as interests and inclusion that are cut up by the lens of representation.[71]

The nexus of the issue is that centring solidarity leads to an entirely different method of engaging with limitations and forms of oppression. Yet, it needs an ethics that focuses on changing lives outside of the institution, rather than in conservative structures that shield transformation. A trans ethics needs to shape space for agency that comes with a humbler approach to one's experience, without sacrificing militancy. If, as Harney and Moten propose, there is a relationship to the institution, it's one of theft – although we have seen Robin Hood join the cops too.[72] So, if we want to keep movements alive, we need to look at forms, relations, and concepts in a different way that helps us create an ethics of transformation.

COMPLICITY, AGAIN

The problem of fragmentation of collectives is a problem of ethics. To explain this, we return to our discussion on complicity and openness that began in Chapter 1. We start from the problem that positionalities make demands on the direction of our attention. Typically, it takes acts of refusal, consciousness-raising, or witnessing violence to step out of the perspective one's positionality shapes on this world. To question this, we discuss the place of one's experience in structures, to propose how to navigate solidarities. One of the tensions we discuss above is the oscillation between making space for agency and experience and working for solidarity in a manner that goes beyond one's direct experience – without falling into managerialism, taking over space, or ignoring the plight of others in favour of 'realistic' possibilities 'that make it better for everyone', where 'everyone' is a bounded group. To do this, we focus on complicity over innocence and oppression, as a method of retaining agency, refusing oppressive structures, and putting our perspective into perspective, so to speak. A focus on complicity means reflection on our positions in structures of power, to face what needs to be refused, what needs to be obstructed and how to lay a claim to the problem that is at hand.[73]

Claiming complicity avoids claiming innocence, which places one outside of the structures of power. Simultaneously, claiming complicity holds space for friction between people. Refusal of power structures alone leaves people isolated and ignores the need to build up the skills that movement work requires, while it bypasses one's implication in the systems that sustain hierarchies.[74] A focus on complicity does not make too much of the difference between 'good and bad' friction but invites practising ethics from where one is, whether it is dealing with everyday friction or supporting people to unlearn bias. Working towards solidarity is one way to move away from fragmentation towards collective action. It refuses the stasis of positionality and replaces it with ethics. This proposition is an inverse of a politics of positionality (similar to identity), where positionality seems to inform how one faces oppression. Marquis Bey remarks that one's positionality might not at all be indicative of whether one is a collaborator with, or an accomplice against, existing structures: 'The weightiness of things formerly known as identities must shift to the ways one deploys oneself in subversion of power, and in alternative relationality'.[75] Bey writes 'Put crassly, you can be racialised Black, identified and identify as a woman or transgender (or both [or all three]) and still do some fucked up shit, still hold steadfast to violent norms'.[76] When modes of violence are what one knows intimately, those modes might resurface in other relations. This can obviously happen with people who are empowered, where the reproduction of familiar modes of engagement is part of the empowerment, but also can equally surface for those who are disempowered, where aligning with hegemonic forms is either demanded or internalised. Hegemony is pernicious, spreading partly through pervasive norms, and inclusion draws us in to participate and to be more *like* the norm. It takes a reflective step, and sometimes support, to break out of such patterns. Therefore, we propose to use positionality to indicate how to investigate which refusals are needed from where one finds oneself, where is one implicated, and which ethics could counter-balance complicities. Trans, viewed as a movement away from an assigned position, implies such non-static positionality as a gendered relationality, but it is radical only insofar as trans manifests as anti-normative actions that support the abolition of hegemonic ways of being.[77]

To think about such an ethics that deals with complicity and non-positionalities, we need to review how institutions function to retain positionalities in stasis. Market forces are racist, sexist, transphobic, xenophobic, and ableist, and institutional in the sense that they are inevitable patterns that are enforced by policy and even in the name of fairness. As we have argued above, rights intend (or pretend) to mediate market forces, which permits a spectacle of inclusion that is nevertheless predicated upon the necessity of exclusion, expropriation, and extraction. Aiming for rights to guarantee normative access suggests a hope for a frictionless environment, in which one has the liberty to individualise oneself, free from constraints (and thus the limitations of identity).[78]

FRICTIONLESS ENVIRONMENTS
AND STRUCTURES OF DOMINATION

As we discussed in Chapter 1, an investment in a frictionless environment is often explained as *white innocence*, which oftentimes leads to a 'smug ignorance' of those who are privileged in this normative order.[79] Such claims to innocence are harmful in their denial of violent structures, or even simply aggressive. In institutional contexts they may emerge as the bourgeois feminine complement to masculine transgressions.[80] In addition to recognising fear as a social force that puts pressure on our relations, we also recognise the desire for 'obnoxious agency' as such a force. Obnoxious agency is the desire for the power to ignore any form of accountability (except perhaps within violent hierarchies). As Christopher Lew proposes to read white supremacy, '[r]ather than an issue of emotion, racism is a way to get rich without overhead, a way to kill without consequence'.[81] The suggestion that racism is driven by fear might, at times, be used to individualise racism, and maintain middle-class arrogance, by staging racism as an emotional problem found in people at the bottom layers of society; but we can recognise fear as the fear for accountability and loss of protection by normative hierarchies.[82] A demand for obnoxious agency can be seen as a demand for some of the power that others hold in a violently hierarchical system, and thus emerges as the demand for the power to exploit in one's immediate surroundings. Fear and obnoxious agency emerge in tandem, as gendered dynamics in the guise of innocence and transgression, which play out to refuse accountability to those (set up to be) closed out from the normative space that binary whiteness protects. Innocence coheres heteronormative feminine virtues – and a claim to innocence signals the willingness to guard dominant norms, showing that the claimant is willing to be subject to them. In this context, masculine transgressions of dominant norms signal that one feels exempt from scrutiny and accountability. Yet, these transgressions are empowered by institutionalised norms.

Deviation from the norm 'invites' punishment that keeps the normative space closed and under hierarchical control. Philomena Essed and Isabel Hoving explain the institutionalised lack of accountability through the disposition of smug ignorance, which can be understood as the effect of denying harmful actions by means of available social power.[83] When there is public awareness of these dynamics, liberal approaches hope that there can be an institutional space, structured by norms, inclusive enough to allow for internal accountability. In this restructure, institutions endeavour to be free from having to consider different, outside perspectives.[84] Liberal spaces thus protect and contain a single order that refuses to engage with different ways of being in the world.[85] This means that inclusion requires that marginalised people adhere to norms and the logics of the existing space, and in this manner inclusion protects the functioning of white patriarchal capitalist organisation.[86] A pervasive, banal and everyday masculinised carelessness and indifference, which is the effect of an over-empowered agency, underwrites a feminised fear that leads to investing in a centralised power – power that will keep such aggressive masculine sociality in check.[87] This tautology is structured by everyday violence, where the potential of patriarchal violence leads to the investment in normative patriarchal organisations, as a form of protection against the transgressive side of patriarchy. Quan understands the resulting paternalism as reflecting an 'addiction to the state' or, as we add, to institutions.[88] This investment in punishment culture plays out on various scales in society – on the personal level and on political levels, where liberals claim to be the bulwarks against the neofascists. Simultaneously, a fear of nonnormative difference, that translates itself as a feminised 'concern', works to close off institutional spaces. This means that requests for inclusion based on innocence and unjust victimisation backfire, by enforcing the power of dominant gendered relations, which cannot hold space for different experiences, ethics, and insights.

On a practical level, we can see this in how the demand for, and implementation of, hate crime legislation is channelled into an investment in punitive cultures. Sarah Lamble lays out that hate crime legislation doesn't make us safer, and the argument that they are 'prevention-driven' is false. Hate crime legislation comes always after the fact, and doesn't prevent aggression *per se*, but adds the threat of severe punishment (as apparently deterrent).[89] Lamble draws attention to the problem that the threshold of proof that the offence was motivated by hate is quite high, and as such is unlikely to tackle the many everyday forms of harassment.[90] The offer of punishment comes in the form of a 'false offer of recognition', by 'tak[ing] the symbolic aspect of recognising harm and channel[ing] it into a punitive response (tougher sentencing) that does little to stop the violence and instead shores up the powers of the carceral state'.[91] It turns organisations that previously worked against criminalisation towards supporting expanding forms of state violence. Lamble summarises this as the promise of violence that is offered as a solution to social anxieties.[92] It offers a distinction between worthy and dangerous citizens, where the latter are staged as the causes of anxiety.

The analysis of contemporary structures of institutional forms shows that inclusion does not function as a *disciplinary* genre of patriarchy. In addition to the directly violent form of patriarchy, Françoise Vergès offers that '(h)eads of State have adopted a "soft", feminist, and humanist patriarchy that contrasts sharply with a vulgar, racist, homophobic, transphobic patriarchy that boasts of "grabbing women by the pussy" and is contemptuous of State institutions'.[93] Authority in revamped 'soft' institutions takes the form of fragmentation of different positions (trans, Black, neurodivergent as differences that need inclusion), rather than grasping command of a single narrative, which people are expected to adhere to. The fragmentation into identity categories that each require bespoke formulas of address is a barrier by management against a combined critique of hierarchies. Dealing with differences in practice is relegated to the shop floor, while management issues top-down policies that structure work. Institutional investment in the structure of organisational forms leaves content (of literature, films, seminars) open, while patriarchy retreats into a control of structure. Content is immobilised in inflexible organisational forms. Liberalism's single order works to hedge against what seems to – from its perspective – be chaos and an overwhelming variety of ways of worlding. Such hedging takes, for instance, a non-reliance on non-institutional organisations, leaving marginalised community-based organisations struggling to connect to institutions. It claims to solve problems by imposing policies that stifle potentiality through metrics, that reinforce hierarchy, and make people individually responsible for their well-being. The aim of such policies is to shape a frictionless space, modelled on an unhindered flow of commodities and labour.[94] Outside of the workplace, a frictionless space structures sociality through money. Neoliberal market thinking is directly translated into social life: individual wants are accommodated by paid services that require no social obligation. In the workplace, 'diversity' is lauded, while work is stripped of collective social life.[95]

Such approaches are partly the cause of a particular form of obnoxious agency that plays out under the guise of 'freedom of speech'. This false freedom is stripped of accountability, in part because it is liberated from responsibility for structures.[96] Taking liberties in speech seems to be a response to the removal of content from patriarchal organisational forms that have retreated into background structure. The defence of social privilege by means of aggressive statements under the guise of 'freedom of speech' is indicative of this shifting social power. The spectre of the 'girl boss' is an effect of the reformation of visibly patriarchal structures as structures of control, which are always presented as 'more objective'. With this suggestion of objectivity, it is no surprise that aggression is channelled through 'freedom of speech', a principle that has become a cloaca of normative resentment. The anxiety and anger of those (still) privileged within the dominant social norms is indicative of the shift from direct power to indirect support. Similarly, in such spaces, policy is bolstered by compliance, through claims to innocence from a position of white heteronormative femininity. While such claims defend dominant norms, challenges to innocence are seen as violent and in need of policing.[97] The content-free approach of organisations bypasses a recognition of duress, while at the same supporting claims towards diversity and objectivity.

Liberal defences of institutional forms block collective knowledge that challenges these organisational approaches. Such defences often rely on refusing contradictions that can, in fact, be complementary and meaningful. The denial of our knowledge, ways of organising and socialising gets used against us, our lives, friends, and spaces where we gather – while these knowledges, including some tensions, form the heart of our social lives. To return here to our plea for openness that ended Chapter 1, such openness first and foremost holds the socialities within, by putting relations before exclusion and order. Thinking with complicity is done in part by claiming to be part of the problem, which means that we claim to be part of the conflicts against duress and domination. Which *part* exactly that is, remains open – but our claim is a refusal to let go of the problem. Through that claim, we refuse innocence, as innocence is made possible by adherence to norms. All this means we don't strive for a frictionlessness. Hierarchies that maintain innocence ignore the friction that sociality is made of. This friction is not solved by being right – as knowledge-driven middle-class approaches would have it – but it is about the possibility of facing ourselves and each other to change how we make worlds together.[98] We are not better than anyone, we are simply the rest. As Mariame Kaba and Kai Cheng Thom discuss, claiming complicity and participation may lead towards a set of abolitionist practices that do not rely on the victim–perpetrator schema, yet requires difficult conversations.[99] Similarly, Stefano Harney and Fred Moten propose that embracing complicity disrupts individuation, which is imposed by institutions. Instead, it allows a collective mode of approaching duress.[100] Complicity in Harney and Moten's understanding takes two different forms: on the one hand it can be the complicity one experiences when one is individualised in an organisation, and on the other hand complicity is the openness one feels in the acknowledgement that one is never sufficient by oneself, and that togetherness is a response against the separation by institutions. This latter kind of complicity is a refusal of being 'good' in the eyes of the empowered, because goodness means to be unthreatening and thus to effectively hinder one's own liberation.[101]

Claiming to be part of the problem ensures that our problems remain collective ones and holds space for collective involvement. A refusal to have problems regulated away requires reflection on agency and positionality. The lens of complicity unravels the perspective on problems from the notions that friction is simultaneously general (your actions are the expression of your positionality in relation to my actions as the translation of my positionality) and individualised (you are solely responsible for your actions), as if friction is the direct expression of an interrelation between two people as the expression of general structures.[102] Complicity goes both ways: it requires facing one's actions *and* being accountable for how one's positionality might inform those actions. As we have discussed, claiming to be part of the problem disallows an escape into liberal innocence, because, to invoke Miss Major and Arthur Rimbaud, we are still here – and that means we won't let the problem go (by, for instance, allowing people to evade their responsibility for a problem), nor will we be removed. In moralist inversions of the structures of duress, it is claimed that (formerly) oppressed *positionalities* offer special moral insights. However, while Blackness and transness can show the way to liberation, as Moten, Bey, and Snorton contend, it is not because of being a generalised category, but because of sociality and resistance that has survived and formed under duress.[103] This contrasts with institutions, because the institution exists to individualise and empower those up the hierarchy, and it is expected that one behaves according to one's place in the hierarchy. The well-known trope of claiming that it is only 'bad apples' that harass, for example, students (or arrestees, or incarcerated people), ensures that structures of duress, precarity, overwork, and power imbalance do not need to be addressed. Complicity reminds us to acknowledge that interrelations are already contextual. For instance, toleration or hierarchy might have structured the actions of the 'bad apple'.

A collective responsibility for practices, including the responsibility to change them, spotlights another way of engaging friction. This shift from individual accountability, with its resonance of calculable and individualised wrongs, to collective responsibility is made possible by the eager claim to complicity.[104] As an example, Gloria Anzaldúa narrates how she entered a conflict at a feminist conference with her knowledge and politics, but despite her experience she found herself in a position where she became implicated in the argument.[105] While it is almost a standard problem that social tensions arise in certain feminist conferences, in contrast to the more usual claims of good intentions and innocence, Anzaldúa has the courage to admit that she became part of the problem. From within positions of hegemonic whiteness, this step is often avoided, or it is translated directly into guilt, innocence, or self-centredness. Reviewing our actions through complicity emphasises entanglement, and highlights how our actions are part of the relations that we are dealing with. Resisting a certain pattern does not set us apart but keeps us part of the situation – this means that we do not critically rise above a situation, but we remain present within it. Openness and entanglement mean that we are *here*, whether we want to be or not.

NO TRANS LIBERATION IN A HOSTILE ENVIRONMENT

The wake of the 2016 Brexit vote, and the upsurge in racist and xenophobic sentiments over the late 2010s and early 2020s, has led to the reconsideration of the UK state from decolonial and anti-colonial perspectives. Amid the intensification of totalitarian policies such as the Hostile Environment, the Police, Crime, Sentencing and Courts Act 2022 and Nationality and Borders Act 2022;[106] and economic, social and physical fallouts of austerity and the coronavirus pandemic, we are in a pivotal moment of reframing our understanding of Britain as empire and its ongoing legacies. Truths regarding how Britain is constituted, the proposed direction of the British nation-state and the conservative/far-right nationalist vision for society have been revealed through the Hostile Environment policies and the 2018 Windrush Scandal. We understand that the logics behind these policies work to uphold white supremacy through forging separability – between people enclosed in norms and those actively marginalised by them. This separability plays out structurally – legally, economically, socially and culturally – from active disenfranchisement through a denial of legal rights, to bureaucratic and/or interpersonal and/or other forms of duress in the workplace or in society, and more casual everyday practices of socially excluding people deemed different from norms. In a context of a white supremacist state, these dynamics of separability primarily work through 'race', the mobilisation of racial grammars, xenophobia and law, whereby cultural difference, in Denise Ferreira da Silva's understanding, is mobilised to 'delimit the reach of the ethical notions of humanity'.[107] In short, separability manifests through structures of the law, economics, hegemonic social norms and cultures, and politics to pronounce *who matters*, and who doesn't. These dynamics draw from histories of coloniality, colonisation and dispossession, slavery and racial capitalism. Today, borders, policing and various forms of incarceration (including immigration detention) play central roles in maintaining separability. In Brexit Britain, anti-blackness and xenophobia in service of white supremacy have trumped even economic logics – with Britain facing a labour shortage significant enough to affect food supplies. While the Home Office creates new tiers, barriers and divisions through the immigration system, this produces a scarcity of agricultural, health, and care workers (the need for this labour was previously filled by migrant workers). Precarity, of temporary or seasonal labour contracts and immigration status, ramps up exploitation of workers and conditions of modern slavery. This is made worse because the promise of Brexit Britain was one of surveillance and friction for those marginalised by their legal status around migration and citizenship, while protecting national resources for white British people.

It is from this current context that Nadine el-Enany encourages us to think of Britain 'as a contemporary colonial space', whereby British colonialism is an 'ongoing project, sustained via the structure of law' and through historical and contemporary immigration laws in particular.[108] As we learn from Kojo Koram, the wealth that enabled the foundations of the British welfare state, including the NHS, in the late 1940s–1950s – the period after World War II and of formal decolonisation – was the wealth of an empire, albeit one in decline.[109] El-Enany argues that the UK's immigration acts across the twentieth and twenty-first centuries, in concert with the border regime and visa requirements, function as 'part of an attempt to control access to the spoils of empire which are located in Britain'.[110] El-Enany continues:

> Britain's borders, articulated and policed via immigration laws, maintain the global racial order established by colonialism, whereby colonised peoples are dispossessed of land and resources. They also maintain Britain as a racially and colonially configured space in which the racialised poor are subject to the operation of internal borders and are disproportionately vulnerable to street and state terror. Britain is thus not only bordered, but also racially and colonially ordered.[111]

El-Enany encourages us to clearly understand that the British state is actively invested in maintaining white supremacy through its laws and policies, which create the conditions for diminished life opportunities – and the diminishment of life itself – for poor Black and Brown people in particular. With reference to the Windrush Scandal and the 2017 Grenfell Tower fire, el-Enany emphasises that amid the legal structures of Britain understood as a colonial space, 'the racialised poor find themselves segregated and controlled, vulnerable to deprivation, exile and death'.[112] The ongoing racial and colonial ordering of Britain produces separability as essential to the functioning of the nation-state – Britain does not cohere without subjecting the racialised poor (including migrants) to policing, surveillance, and terror. These legal structures perpetuate logics that forge divisions and separations in who is entitled to the resources of the British state – both those that are managed by the state to those that are often provided privately – across healthcare, housing, welfare, education, work, and travel.

In a context that promotes rights as the alternative to exclusion, we as marginalised people need to understand clearly what neo-liberal multicultural political endeavours are promising for 'us'. Indeed, el-Enany, alongside thinkers across critical race studies and Indigenous studies, and in concert with queer theorists, encourages us to be cautious of pursuing a politics of recognition, as recognition makes little attempt to unsettle a racially and colonially ordered state. She writes: 'Recognition-based approaches to migrant solidarity that centre the inclusion of racialised people within the colonial state have the effect of obscuring and legitimising the colonial structures underlying British immigration, asylum and nationality laws'.[113] Appeals to recognition tend to function along the axis of a single issue, without interrogation of the structure, nor a disruption of the logics of ordering. To interrogate structures risks undermining one's inclusion within them and is 'unacceptable' to a politics based on respectability. El-Enany emphasises the conditionality of recognition, buffered by the (often extensive) bureaucratic processes around visas, asylum claims and the border, which both legitimise a colonial state and use the law to deny racialised people access to the state's resources.[114] To be aware of these structures of xenophobic and racialising exclusion when developing a trans politics, offers two key insights: first, inclusion for some will always be only conditional – when social structures function to exclude and police access for others, what is given at one time, can easily be taken away at another time. Second, economic structures work to guard the unequal division of resources, and that a trans politics that does not address this, will not be working for liberation, but for the entrenchment of these divisions of separability.

MOVEMENTS, RELATIONS, AND COLLECTIVITY

To conclude this chapter, we look at how separability is at play in social life. We tie this to our arguments on institutional policy, borders, and the expressions of anti-trans and racist imaginaries in contemporary politics. Normative and routinised social skills are related to positions in social forms, although they are not a homogenous set of actions.[115]

Adherence to norms can make possible one's inclusion in a specific space, while these social routines can at that same time concretely reproduce divisions of class, gender, racialisation, ableism, and more. At other times, norms may also reproduce more localised dynamics such as workplace hierarchies, housing privileges, or institutional belonging. The politics of inclusion means that expectations of who occupies certain positions can shift, and the attendant liberal hope is for a shift in ethics. We have discussed how disciplinary power, which made strong claims about social roles, transforms into a softer form with tight organisational control (soft patriarchy). This also means that changing expectations around positionalities becomes an integral part of institutional (re)forms, when previously, social markers had meant definite social placement. These changes come with a demand for a modicum of skill in 'diversity work', and are met with active resistance by the right (animating their entitlement, fear, anxieties, hatred of difference, and obnoxiousness). When we do see a shift in ethics, people become more adept at managing their expectations on fulfilling who occupies which role. However, the hope that inclusion will introduce a non-exploitative ethics is rarely fulfilled, as the control of structures guarantees a continuation of patriarchy, albeit by a larger range of people occupying a larger set of positions. The display of morality (however sincere) that inclusion affords is only possible through the stabilisation of hierarchy that the institutionalisation of power generates. It doesn't address how hierarchy creates oppression – so perhaps we can see inclusion as an aesthetics, which prevails through visibility, rather than an ethics.[116] Inclusion shifts everyday atmospheres within organisations, giving a new flair to existing relations of control.

To hold ourselves against the onslaught of (trans)misogyny, and forms of racist violence inflicted upon the world by patriarchy, we refuse the unfreedoms of choice and individualised power. We work towards a freedom in relation, that can be said to be a movement away from an unchosen starting point but is made together. Echoing Harney and Moten, it is collectivity, an unfree sociality, in which we are held together. We have proposed neither to think of possibility through the overarching platform of an institution (perhaps a nation), nor through the possessive individualism of personal choice (where *you* get it *your way*); but instead, as part of a collectivity, we aim to reimagine institutional, individualist, and possessive agency. We hold on to each other, refuse the grasp of power, to emerge in collectives and social forms. This is not freedom of speech, nor freedom of choice, but a *freedom in relation*. Liberation through relation may be marked by what Moten and Harney call indebtedness – without each other and the movement struggle that comes before and is to come, and that exists now, we wouldn't be here. By nurturing collectivities that are outside of dominant social forms, an openness can exist, that doesn't depend on stable forms of life. Mindful of María Lugones' warnings that *nonnormative* collectives also use purification to control their inner workings[117] – that they can police right and wrong, push people out, and demand 'proper' behaviour, seeking perhaps 'their own' virtuousness or simply respectability. Instead, if we hold on to each other, and work to remain in relation, including honing the skills that nurture collectivity, forms of living emerge that can avoid getting ossified in 'proper' forms, and remain open.[118] Through openness and refusal, we figure out how to change and transform together, knowing that frictions will emerge and that it will get messy.

When sociality is structured around openness, dominant forms need to be refused too. Marquis Bey formulates it as follows: '[t]he prefixal *anarcho-* describes a world-making, a creative imaginative praxis reliant upon a pervasive *un-* that erects more than it destroys'.[119] Abolition as a mode of world-making doesn't intend to simply remove harmful and violent structures – abolitionist practices come with an expansive remaking of alternatives, of worlds that emerge directly between us and those who act with us.[120] Compared to institutional inclusion, where there is at best minimal change in the organisation of its hierarchies; the anarchic needs to tend to equity – if it intends to dismantle social hierarchies and its twin technology, command.[121] As we will discuss in Chapter 5, such a praxis blooms when based on an ethics of generosity.

While – also on the left – the desire persists for a leader or someone to make the world right, abolition emphasises the direct transformative quality of working collectively, and abolition itself as a politic is nourished through making space for people's insights, imaginations, and needs. Abolition works by embracing a multitude of experiences, even if working together coalesces around the commonalities in difference, confronting pressures that are urgent. Even when we are not directly in the line of fire, we know that to dismantle structures of duress will ultimately benefit all of us, provided we are actively unspooling separability. In this coming together, the experiences of institutionalisation and its concurrent harms need witnessing, working against, and growing sensitivity to inform one's ethics.[122]

Transition, transformation, and trans practices put ensouled bodyminds in motion – through physical space, social circles, cities or countries; through the change that emerges through our bodyminds; and through shifts in how we advocate or affirm our genders in our lives. We learn new ways to move, dance, speak, describe, and joke; we find new means to protest and resist. In such activities, the ethics that emerge require their own balancing act. If we frame exclusion – individually, or as a community – as exceptional and narrate it primarily through a trope of unjust victimisation, without understanding its entanglements within systems that harm and obstruct the lives of many, we risk a bourgeois trans position which can be easily met and demobilised by a politics of institutional inclusion. As we have argued, entanglements should not only be understood in a 'classical' sense of complicity, but also through our proposed conceptualisation that being part of a world makes one responsible for it. Victimisation, in contrast, explains one's position through innocence and detachment. A trans movement that primarily focuses on its unjust exclusion has a tendency to see itself as frictionless, as also does the managerial realm itself. This idea has been criticised for ignoring a complexity of duress, in favour of a self-referential politics that sacrifices solidarity.[123]

Trans refusal as movement can be understood through Harney and Moten as 'collective self-possession', where collectivity means that we remain incomplete together.[124] Incompleteness means we are never anything without each other. While some of us might be messy, we learn from the mess – sometimes, we learn about our own hang-ups and get confronted with our desires for a certain kind of relation. This means that forms can remain flexible and become spaces for becoming, emergence, and change. Through movements, we create space for collective resistance, connecting to our surroundings, and for collective flourishing.

4

Medical institutions, collective care

INTRODUCTION

In the last chapter we discussed the troubled entanglements of identities with institutions and borders, and how certain forms of inclusion demobilise movements and leave people disempowered. We highlighted the traps of identity, where leading with either social categories or our individual experiences of limitations generalises those very identities and seemingly makes them issues of knowledge, rather than what they also are: practices and ways of making new relations. Trans genders do not need to be legible and can hover on the edges of understanding, in part because they do not need to become fixed. Instead, trans might be seen as a kinetic movement out of the confines of what is known, led by pleasure and even eroticism, as we discussed in Chapter 1.[1] Trans comes out from under the debris of normative genders and queer insights, but is also more than that – trans becomes forms of coming together that allow for exploration and making meaning beyond what is already given. As we have shown, trans' radical potential entails creating relations that make it possible for something new to emerge. Such activity is always collective activity, that, as Travis Alabanza writes, 'is *for us*, baby'.[2] The plural is the message – contra individualising tropes, trans is never singular, transness emerges collectively, and makes collectivity. Sometimes trans relationalities are sufficient to give form to one's life, although this is not always the case. Medical treatments, hormones, or surgeries can support embracing one's bodily being, connection in one's relationships, and shifting our ensouled bodyminds from one way of being in the world to other ways of worlding. This leads us to the next confrontation: if we cannot shrug off institutions because medical needs play a part in trans exploration, what do we do then? In this chapter we look at medical institutions and the troubled role they play in trans lives. We question how care is given, sometimes turned into violence and hostility, and often simply inadequate.

We have discussed elsewhere how neoliberalism emphasises individual responsibility for one's well-being.[3] This fundamental trope of neoliberalism is, however, also impossible. Amidst hostile environments and atmospheres of violence, one cannot individually care for one's own well-being as well-being depends on social life. This includes resistance to violence and duress, and navigating together the institutions that are responsible for it. Violence – from institutions, or a hostile social world – can be direct; and sometimes violence is experienced indirectly – not targeted at an individual, but at their friend or acquaintance.[4] Sometimes violence is impersonal and doled out so widely that everyone in a group is affected. One example of this is Stop and Search, an everyday violence that is directed generically at young Black, Asian, and minority ethnic men and children.[5] Medical violence in Gender Clinics is another example of violence that is impersonal – the hostile approach to trans people typical of clinics, within which psychiatrists retain the power to sign off on or deny us treatment, makes interactions almost unanimously anxiety-inducing.

Healthcare is integral to a politics of trans liberation. While politicised trans communities have long since moved past a limited understanding of transness as predicated on medical transition, accessing, negotiating, and receiving medical treatment remains a key material and political struggle for many of us. However, as Ruth Pearce discusses in her book on trans healthcare, literature produced by medical practitioners on trans health is largely focused on transition, at the expense of addressing wider issues around trans health.[6] This has the effect of limiting gender-variant experience, in the medical sphere, as 'a very particular, conditional form of trans possibility', and furthermore of eliding other experiences of trans people that function as comorbidities.[7] This includes risks of alcohol and substance abuse, mental distress, self-harm, HIV infection rates, experiencing violence, alongside 'significantly higher prevalence of autistic spectrum conditions' among non-binary, genderqueer and trans people. Pearce, reading Sandy Stone and Joanne Meyerowitz, nonetheless emphasises the agency of trans people in affecting the access to treatment and 'the transsexual medical model' itself in the twentieth century – as our 'active efforts' in the difficult task of 'educat[ing] health professionals' has enabled our embodied existences, even in the context of medical gatekeeping and pathologisation.[8]

By healthcare, we mean both healthcare directly related to gender transition (referred to as 'gender-affirming healthcare'), *and* the healthcare across all areas of medicine sought out by trans and non-binary people. In these more general spaces, our senses of self may be grated by the cis- and heteronormativity, whiteness, misogyny, and ableism often ingrained into medical provisions, or into the ideas of what a 'healthy body' is or looks like. The cisnormativity of many medical services – framing provisions within the gender binary – creates additional barriers to access for non-binary people, or pressures us to conform to gender norms.[9] Sites of healthcare include formal institutions within the medical profession (hospitals and clinics), more community-focused organisations and groups (directly connected to the medical profession or not), formal social care, and the formal and informal relations that make up social life such as receiving care from friends or family members (offering paracetamol, tending a wound, cooking and cleaning when one is ill). By thinking through a wide scope of trans healthcare – where even gender-affirming care may involve procedures that both trans and non-trans bodyminds may undergo – we can connect across struggles that may typically be considered separate. Struggles for reproductive justice and assisted reproduction, HIV/AIDS prevention and treatments, harm reduction services, 'gender-responsive' specialist treatments (such as cancer treatments), better support for neurodiversity in and beyond healthcare, and unsettling essentialist gender norms across areas of healthcare provision, are all struggles trans people have stakes within.

CLINICS AND THE POWER OF BINARIES

Conservative, ableist, and patriarchal norms, which form the sex/ gender binary, proclaim: 'this is how your body will be, this is how it will grow throughout your life'; 'this is what your body does or can do, this is what it is prohibited from doing'; 'this is your role in sexual reproduction'; 'these are the forms of care you must perform for men, women, and children'; 'this is the degree of freedom you are permitted with your body' (in regards to sex, in regards to body modifications ranging from hair removal to tattoos to cosmetic surgeries, et al.); 'these are the degrees of subservience you must adhere to'. Allegiance to embodying the norms of gender has long determined how coherent one appears to the wider social world, and how one falls into the orders of racial capitalism. Transness unsettles the coherence of how gender norms are embodied, as we take flight and manifest gender on, in and through other ways of embodiment and of using one's body (expressively, materially, sexually, reproductively). Feminisms ranging from conservative to (neo)liberal to progressive may challenge the terms of gender norms and the prescriptions/proscriptions delineated by them – although, for institutions and bureaucracy within the liberal public sphere, gender coherence seemingly remains a condition of citizenship. Indeed, the legal recognition of transness (discussed in Chapter 3) is usually premised on one's gender change within the binary as being 'permanent', that one is 'living full time in their acquired gender'.[10] This legal permanence in gender may be undergirded by the medicalisation and psychiatrisation of gender, whereby transition between the 'two' sexes is framed as a permanent journey in one direction.

One institution that trans and non-binary people are confronted with is the Gender Clinic (Gender Identity Clinic or GIC), which in the context of the UK has a monopoly of power over provision and access to gender-affirming healthcare. Outside of private and collective healthcare, the Gender Clinic maintains authority over deciding if one is entitled to gender-affirming treatment in accordance with diagnostic criteria, what treatments or surgeries one will receive and when (according to treatment or surgical pathways), and how long one will have to wait to receive treatment. Trans liberation entails a more equitable access to healthcare, and moreover for *depathologised treatment* that doesn't reinforce gender norms, without the threat of it being denied if one doesn't abide by the strict regulations of the Gender Clinic. While there have been pushes to increase funding to NHS trans healthcare – as seen in Scotland in 2020 – we need funding and resources that directly improve access, reduce hierarchies of power, and make room for agency, rather than simply expanding the resources of the Gender Clinic. Expanding the clinic's resources will maintain psychiatric and state power over trans and non-binary bodies.[11]

When I, Mijke, came to the Gender Clinic in the early 2000s, there were already waiting lists. The situation was partly institutionalised: we had to wait six months, to make sure we wouldn't change our minds. This should have been warning enough. All of us were there to change our bodyminds, after all, but that was not the going medical paradigm. Medical thought at the time was that trans people had a differently gendered mind and 'normal' body, and this 'mental problem' could only be solved by adapting the body – via Hormone Replacement Therapy (HRT) and surgeries.[12] Meanwhile, gender studies, especially under the influence of Judith Butler, proposed the idea that one's mind imposes how the body is perceived.[13] Trans people are often hovering between these ideas, partly depending on whether they have had academic training, and when they had it. Despite gender studies departments' approaches to the Cartesian dilemma of minds reading bodies, trans people insist quite regularly that bodies are different from minds.[14] As we have made the case throughout this book, there is no split, but we live through ensouled bodies with their immersed minds, with ripple effects of actions and medical interventions in all directions, and partly by exploring new ways of living life. The immersed perception of life is the fundamental difference between the pathologising approach of the Gender Clinic to trans people and the approach of trans people to themselves.[15] Gender is personal and shared at the same time. It is relational, but also (at times) deeply felt (like Judith Butler suggests) or simply hovering around when you pay attention to it, to gender as a system being something that needs to be escaped time and time again, which Marquis Bey is working through.[16]

To make some sense of this tension between the Gender Clinic and trans people, we will turn to a quote by Carl Schmitt. Carl Schmitt is a fascist philosopher, and as such has not much to say about trans people, but offers some insights about the workings of the Gender Clinic. If we accept that gender is both shared and personal, Schmitt's statement that 'who guards something, owns it' makes sense with regard to the condescending approach of psychologists, psychiatrists, and clinicians at the clinic.[17] While trans people are renewing gendered cultures, opening up space for exploration or escape, clinicians are guarding the appropriate norms and forms of gendering. It also works to make clear who apparently owns gender: they do, not trans people. In the relatively short time that one spends in the clinic – an hour a month or quarter during the screening process, or meeting endocrinologists, or a week when receiving surgery – staff at the clinics focus on containing the gendered overspill. These condensed moments are rear-guard actions by clinicians defending normative gender from escapee trans people; although, we do most of the work out of their sight anyway – and both parties know it. This contrasts a Foucauldian approach that would argue that the clinic disciplines trans people.[18] But the clash in the clinic may be better perceived as wrestling for ownership of gender from clinicians, with trans people running off with the fun part of it anyway. If we look at norms not through their content, but through who claims the power to guard them, we can see how gendered norms are dynamic (they change), while power stays in the same hands. Similar to management – who enforce control of organisational structures, while leaving the content of those structures open – the work of guardians of the norm is a structural protection of power. The scrutiny of trans people is done regardless of the awareness that norms are dynamic and changeable: in our lifetimes everybody can see norms changing between generations. The stakes in the clinic's ownership of gender, versus exploration and liberating gender from the confines of normative control, are significant.

THE STAKES OF TRANS HEALTHCARE

The above discussion highlights the way in which trans promotes a cultural shift. In contrast to what clinicians might expect, trans is not about 'knowing who you are'; indeed, people of all genders often do not know this, which is okay. Knowledge is less important than activity, and often in trans experience, we have to throw ourselves into the unknown: come out and see who responds well and who doesn't; take hormones and see what will happen; figure out how to live, re-acquaint oneself with one's desires and needs; or figure out how to navigate pressures, dangers, and alliances, and imagine (im)possible futures, often by sheer force of will and the love of other trans people. The hurdle of announcing oneself to the world is merely a moment, but it's a huge shift to re-organise life – no matter how small one thinks it will be. Indeed, it is in our vulnerable moments – when we are in need of treatment – that we come to Gender Clinics. In this vulnerability, we are exposed to the intense pressures of medical institutions, and may get caught up in having to prove ourselves worthy or 'correct' to the clinic. Yet, there are ways in which the harms can be reduced, by institutions offering alternatives to pathologisation and the centring normative embodiment, as well as by the collective work of caring for each other.

Affirmative healthcare is just one aspect of what public health scholars and professionals describe as the social determinants of health. Social determinants link together the social, economic, geographic, political, and micropolitical to understand how they affect access to health care and to 'health' as understood as 'wellness, strength and stability.'[19] Writing in *Trans Bodies, Trans Selves*, Nick Gorton and Hilary Maia Grubb also describe the importance of 'stable employment, a safe home and environment [...] access to healthy food choices, and opportunities to exercise', alongside the availability of 'trans and gender-expansive-competent and affirming health care' in a broad sense.[20] The authors note that trans and gender-expansive people are less likely to have 'routine' healthcare needs met, such as 'routine vaccinations for preventable illnesses, treatment of chronic health conditions [...] routine screenings for diseases such as breast, cervical and colon cancer', describing how '[m]any of us have delayed or avoided healthcare and health maintenance screenings because of negative interactions within the healthcare system or fears of such'.[21]

At the core of trans and non-binary healthcare struggles is the relationship between one's ensouled bodymind and the social context, relations, and networks one is situated amidst. While the embodied experiences of transness have long been pathologised by psychiatrists and medical professionals, in practice our embodied experiences have lasting personal and social effects.[22] Experiences of dissonance, dysphoria, depression, discomfort with certain aspects of our bodyminds, or how our embodiment is reflected in ourselves, and how we are received, read, gendered, or misgendered in wider social interactions, affect our everyday senses of moving into and through the world. Between, say, dysphoria, a lack of self-confidence, a disparate and dispersed social world, and the interplay of the structural and social effects of transphobia, transmisogyny, and other forms of oppression, one's opportunities for work or for material stability may be limited. It's common, for instance, in trans communities to find one's life on hold while one is waiting for healthcare to make one's existence less challenging, draining, or laborious (an experience that might be common for non-trans people too). Trans and queer communities and collectives provide energy, skills, and encouragement to live on and express oneself in the face of limited opportunities or delays in accessing life-affirming healthcare – to eke out life, nonetheless. The struggle for trans healthcare is a struggle for more life, toward self-realisation through one's bodymind as a deep need and desire, for possibility in self-expression.

SMASHING THE POWER OF GIC

Like any marginalised group trying to meet their health needs through recourse to the medical establishment, trans people have long since shared information regarding services and provisions, treatments and technologies, and embodied experiences, regarding transition and broadly accessing healthcare. This is in a context of a long history of the medical gatekeeping of gender-affirming healthcare, primarily by psychiatrists, and the framing of such healthcare through medical pathologies. Trans activists and organisations appealed for the depathologisation of trans healthcare, with old pathologies such as 'gender identity disorder' being reformed to reduce objectifying elements of their character in the most recent edition of *DSM*. In the last five years, the depathologisation of gender incongruence has been formalised in the *International Classification of Diseases* (*ICD-11*, 2019) and, in 2022, by the World Health Organisation (WHO), with WPATH's Standards of Care (Eighth edition) published that year.[23] However, as TGEU notes, while '[t]rans identities are no longer pathologised and being trans is not a psychiatric condition', in the EU 'many countries still require a psychiatric diagnosis to access trans-specific healthcare'.[24] In the UK, reform is an ongoing project that ensures psychiatrists maintain power within Gender Identity Clinics, by having the final say on who gets gender-affirming treatment (such as voice training, hair removal, hormones, surgeries), and when. In addition, surgeons often still require letters of clinical sign-off from psychiatrists for gender-affirming procedures. Here, psychiatrists ultimately judge our gender presentations (how masculine or feminine one presents oneself, according to one's chosen gender), the situations of our lives, jobs, and relationships (do we have work, do we have heteronormative or homonormative partners or children, are we transitioning in 'settled' or precarious contexts), alongside our public markers of transition (such as legally changing one's name, being out at work), our needs and desires for our bodyminds, and the degrees of distress that we (have) experience(d). The exceptions are in the handful of NHS pilot schemes, working with a variety of organisations to provide more 'holistic' care, in London, Manchester, Merseyside, and the East of England; and in the everyday healthcare support offered by trans-affirmative health clinics in London and Brighton. The 2024 Cass Report on Gender Identity Services for children and young people in England, which proposes to recentre the power of GICs in regional mental healthcare units, is the latest example of the protection of psychiatric power, in this case over the needs of trans youth.[25]

At the time of writing, the situation with the Gender Clinics is dire. Waiting lists for first appointments for adults at the NHS Gender Clinics vary between one and seven years, with an average of 3¾ years.[26] In July 2023, there were 13,740 people on the waiting list at the Tavistock and Portman GIC in London – the main Gender Clinic in London – with approximately a five-year wait for first appointments.[27] The experience of excessively long wait times for gender-affirmative care is itself distressing,[28] and to describe these waiting times as 'murderous' is not a mere figure of speech. The excessive waiting times faced by Alice Litman – a trans woman from London – contributed to a 'decline' in her health that led to her taking her own life in 2022, aged 20.[29] At the time of her death, Alice had been waiting 1,023 days for gender-affirming treatment; the inquest into her death found that all the services involved in her care were 'underfunded and insufficiently resourced'.[30] Outside the context of gender-affirming treatment, dysphoria and distress regarding one's body are typically understood as experiences requiring prompt treatment as they are debilitating. Although, failures by the local mental health trust treating Sophie Gwen Williams – a trans woman who co-founded the trans collective and mutual aid group We Exist in London – coupled with the excessive waiting times of GICs, had such a 'devasting' effect on Sophie that she took her own life in 2021, aged 28.[31]

As we write elsewhere,

> Our access to healthcare is restricted on the grounds of 'cost effectiveness', while our physical and mental health is deemed a 'personal responsibility', rather than the responsibility of any institutions we interact with, or which fail to provide us with healthcare.[32]

Being forced to wait such excessively long times – especially in the early years of one's life – can be understood as a form of what Dean Spade names 'administrative violence'.[33] The delay, or failure, of bureaucracy to perform its 'duty of care' is experienced as mental and embodied distress; this violence negatively impacts one's everyday life and experience of the world – amplified when trans visibility is met with harm and abuse in the external world. Furthermore, it functions as a disciplinary tool – one must, first, wait patiently before being received as a 'good patient' by the Gender Clinic; those who go private or rogue may be dismissed or discharged. In addition, trans people sometimes end up arguing, especially online, that – in the context of minimal resources that by no means serve everyone – one should wait one's turn on these brutal waiting lists. The lack of resources allocated to trans healthcare – the limited allocation of funding for healthcare, the sparse development of trans-competent provisions, the limited availability of treatments on the NHS (including those widely available privately), alongside the costs of pursuing education in medicine or nursing and the low wages of nurses – is a form of what Ruth Wilson Gilmore calls 'organised abandonment', whereby political decisions are made on where and how to spend public money, and on the racial geographies of where those resources are placed and where they pass over. As Gleeson and Hoad write, 'The GIC system was always a means of state discipline and managed deprivation'.[34] Non-binary people who desire transition-related healthcare may face additional delays, or have their treatment refused.

The exceptionalisation of trans people, which directs us to the Gender Clinic as our 'only option' for treatment, sidelines the fact that many of the treatments we pursue could easily be accessed through GPs (and are accessible for non-trans people via GPs). This ranges from HRT to blood tests (to check hormone levels, liver function, etc.), to hair removal, voice coaching, and more. The need for these treatments to be signed off by psychiatrists at the Gender Clinic reinforces pathologisation, and the difficulty of accessing the clinic itself leaves us to pursue other options. Although, GPs also need to do the work of learning about trans healthcare – trans and non-binary people have often had to educate our GPs ourselves, sharing protocols such as the WPATH Standards of Care with them.

Trans people who are incarcerated also face additional problems, given challenges of accessing legal services, materials, and opportunities for gender affirmation, and the practical difficulties of being out and expressing one's gender when inside prisons. In the UK, there is a general principle that incarcerated people are 'entitled to receive the same quality of care in prison as you would expect to receive outside of prison from the NHS'. A 2022 survey of trans prisoners by the Bent Bars Project emphasised that access to healthcare in prison is 'poor and inconsistent'.[35] This included the deferral of promised appointments, delays of 2+ years in communication, a lack of information on medical needs, and bias in treatment. One trans person undertook two hunger strikes to be put in contact with a GIC.[36] If able to access a GIC, incarcerated trans people face additional judgement due to the stigma of criminalisation, the limitations on gender self-expression in prison, and face slower-than-typical treatment timelines, alongside the same troubles as the rest of us.[37] Discussing the American context, Jaclyn Diaz writes 'getting reliable gender-affirming care in prison seems to often come only after threats of lawsuits or an all-out legal fight. Prisons that do provide gender-affirming care can often still be inconsistent, regardless of policies on the books'.[38]

Another major problem is the idea that the GIC provides counselling for trans people – to support our mental health during transition, or in the context of any of the harm or fallout that we might experience while transitioning (e.g. transphobia in family, workplace, social or other institutional contexts). It's commonly raised that trans and non-binary people experience high rates of mental distress – a 2018 survey produced by Stonewall UK reports that 70% of non-binary people and 67% of trans people surveyed had experienced depression, 71% of trans people had experienced anxiety, and that 50% of non-binary people and 46% of trans people had had suicidal thoughts in the previous year.[39] A problem is a lack of concrete attention and resource towards the social and material conditions that undermine our mental health. Some GICs provided highly limited counselling services; given the lack of trust many of us rightly have in the clinics,[40] this may also affect the usefulness of the sessions – especially in the context where mental health, disability, and neurodiversity are often used by psychiatrists as reasons to delay access to transition-related healthcare. It is noted that trans people have poorer access to health services in general, experiencing discriminatory remarks and inappropriate questioning in attempts to access services, which leads to avoiding services and treatment, and lower satisfaction with services in the event of access.[41] The fact that disclosing any mental health diagnosis that one may have been given, or that one experiences mental distress, can lead to delays or refusal of access to gender-affirming healthcare can leave trans and non-binary people having to make a choice between which forms of healthcare are more important to them, leaving one to advocate for oneself along a singular access of need – i.e. to pursue one form of healthcare at a time. In a classic example of what is colloquially referred to as the trans broken arm syndrome, one of the authors was once referred to an orthopaedist, due to having joint pain related to a sprained ankle. On the referral letter, transsexuality was listed as one of the possible causes of joint inflammation. To have some relationship to being transsexual makes life particularly complicated in the case of mental health, in spite of the WHO's depathologisation of transsexuality. While the crisis in trans healthcare around waiting times and a lack of provisions is a key cause of our collective mental distress, it's by no means the *only* cause of distress.

The GIC system is far from improving – GICs remain chronically under-resourced, despite the excessive waiting times and the increase in the number of people seeking gender-affirming healthcare. A 2021 study on experiences of navigating GICs 'found little evidence of trans people experiencing better quality of care' when comparing recent experiences to those of 10–15 years ago.[42] Pathologisation and the gatekeeping of treatment will not stop without the decentring of psychiatry in trans-specific healthcare, and thus the power of psychiatrists (or psychologists in the Netherlands) over trans people and our bodyminds. Trans healthcare does not require institutionalised control. We need more access to, and availability of treatment, this needs to be free from psychiatry. As the WHO's depathologisation shows, monitoring hormone levels can be left with endocrinologists, and surgeries with surgeons. Although surgeons, too, need to be challenged on their use of pathology and their fatphobia – the differential demands placed on trans and non-binary people accessing surgery is also a potential site of feminist solidarity over sexism, sanism, and fatphobia. With the GIC functioning as it is, it is an open question for its service users (and those of us trying to access it) whether we would be better off without it – but what is clear is that we need *actually affirmative* trans healthcare.

TRANS YOUTH

Healthcare provisions for trans youth under the age of 18 are currently also highly limited. In the UK, the few Gender Clinics that provide services to younger people (formerly the Tavistock in London and still the Sandyford in Glasgow) have extensive waiting lists. Following the 2024 Cass Review, trust in these services has dropped significantly, as the Review has led to the ceasing of provisions for puberty blockers for the small number of trans teens who had previously had access to them (which was less than 100 people) in England and Scotland.[43] NHS England is, at the time of writing, commissioning new regional centres for health services for trans and non-binary young people, alongside two 'Phase 1' services in London and Manchester; current service specifications propose that mental health professionals play a more active role in a more 'holistic, multidisciplinary approach' to care for trans and gender-expansive youth and children.[44] LGBTQ+ organisations have raised concerns that such approaches may lead to further pathologisation and gatekeeping of trans and gender-expansive people under 18, especially of neurodiverse and autistic people; may employ medical and psychological staff who lack specialist training in working with trans people, or of the experiences and issues trans people face; and may lead to further delays in treatment (in the context of extensive waiting times) which could entail additional mental distress; and that the proposals place a strong emphasis on psychological and psychosocial support (or intervention), which could dovetail as a form of conversion therapy, in spite of NHS England's commitment to the Memorandum of Understanding on Conversion Therapy.[45]

Gender-affirmative provisions have been the subject of recent legal cases pursued by transphobic feminists to undermine the ability of trans teens under 16 to consent to receiving treatment by challenging Gillick competency as defined in UK law.[46] Despite both medical research and claims from trans and non-binary people regarding the positive outcomes of the use of puberty blockers, new policies severely limit prescribing these to minors even if they are still used for the medical needs of non-trans children. In the words of Gendered Intelligence, 'It's unethical to force a group of people to submit to research in order to get healthcare, and it could stop young people from getting essential support at a vulnerable time.'[47] Within the toxic public discourse on the subject of gender-affirmative healthcare for trans youth, the needs and experiences of trans youth are easily elided under the guise of 'concerns'. To be caught up in distress regarding the development of one's own body during puberty, of how one's body is changing or growing, when one's peers are coming of age as teenagers, is disruptive to education, working, having a childhood or adolescence, living one's life. Blanket claims that trans youth under 16 or 18 will face 'enormous difficulty' to meet the threshold consent to (reversible) treatment under Gillick competency,[48] or that puberty blockers and hormones are medical treatments that in the context of trans youth specifically 'warrant separate legal provision' – with which Court of Appeal ruling on *Bell v Tavistock* (2021) and various legal experts *disagree*[49] – elide the reasons why trans and gender non-conforming youth desire or claim to need such treatment in the first place. In addition, the idea of a separate *legal provision* in order for trans youth to access medical treatments is discriminatory. In their ruling on *Bell v Tavistock*, the Court of Appeal made it clear that 'there was nothing in the nature or effects of puberty blockers that would justify drawing a distinction between them and the provision of contraceptives', and that in the 1980s – when Gillick was decided – the idea of young people accessing contraceptives was, in the Court of Appeal's words, also 'highly controversial in a way that is now hard to imagine.'[50]

Alongside excruciating waits to access treatment through the Gender Clinic, trans youth face additional distress from the lack of knowledge regarding clinical options from healthcare providers – as Matthew Carlile notes in his sociological research with trans youth, a lack of knowledge in Child and Adolescent Mental Health Teams (CAMHS) and in schools is a cause of 'great mental distress' for young trans people.[51] Speaking to both trans young people and children, and to parents, Carlile notes an 'overarching sense' of 'dissatisfaction, frustration, and distress [that] both parents and children or young people felt with healthcare providers – both primary carers and gatekeeper referrers such as GPs and CAMHS, and the specific gender-focused GIDS provision itself'.[52]

Furthermore, in their research interviewing parents of trans children (under 11) accessing healthcare through the Gender Clinic, Cal Horton details how parents often found the clinic 'non-affirmative' in its approach.[53] Parents described how clinicians seemed focused on looking for a 'cause' of a child's transness, through psychoanalytic methods focused on family history, with one participant describing clinicians as 'looking for ways to discredit our child'.[54] Horton details how

A majority (but not all) parents [interviewed] encountered trans negative attitudes at UK Gender Services, especially when attending with younger trans children. Many clinicians inferred (or stated) that a trans child growing up to be a trans adult was a negative, undesirable and avoidable outcome.[55]

Parents described the questions they received in family assessments as 'intrusive and irrelevant', 'insensitive and inappropriate', and 'judgemental, pathologising & outdated'.[56]

SELF-MEDDING

Given the limited provisions of gender-affirming healthcare on the NHS and the chronic underfunding of the NHS, many trans folks make the choice to administer their own gender-affirming medication. Such practices, commonly described as self-medding, entail acquiring medication from private sources, sharing knowledge regarding sources, dosages, and methods of administering medications from within trans communities. This dovetails with practices of harm reduction – sharing information regarding how to use medications as safely as possible, testing bloodwork, and the medications themselves, to ensure bodies and drugs are functioning as they ought to. While this involves risk, self-medding also reclaims agency under material conditions that actively disempower trans people (re: the Gender Clinic), in a context where trans and non-binary people have few options – either wait years for treatment or pursue private means, including moving to another country. Taking risk is no small act, even if trans lives are fraught with everyday forms of risk simply by existing in the world. Given the extent of the psychological/bodily and social difficulties around gender dysphoria, self-medding saves lives. As Gleeson and Hoad write, self-medding entails 'acts of resistance to a system that under-provides skilled treatment as a matter of course.'[57]

Self-medding in trans communities is by no means the first time LGBTQI+ people have taken medical care into their own hands. Between feminist healthcare and queer responses to the HIV/AIDS epidemic, LGBTQI+ history is also replete with examples of collective healthcare. A recent, UK example, can be found with PRePster/I Want PReP Now, whereby since 2010, community activists worked to source highly effective medications that can prevent HIV transmission. PRePster's community-built infrastructure sourced drugs from India, where they can be produced off patent, and distributed the medications (primarily in the UK) to people who were at risk of contracting HIV. This was prior to the licensing of these medications in the UK – at the same time, activists were advocating for their licensing and availability on the NHS, which led to successful legal battles by the National AIDS Trust for PReP and other medications preventative of HIV infection to be available on the NHS – although there is currently varied access depending on where one lives within the UK.[58] PRePster's strategies echoed those of ACT-UP – the AIDS Coalition to Unleash Power, an organisation constituted through international chapters, founded in the late 1980s, that advocated for better treatment for (and of) people who are or were HIV+ by medical providers, government, state, religion, and the media. Reflecting on the shift in cultures around using PReP among gay men, trans and non-trans women who have sex with men or other trans people, and who are at risk of HIV+ infection – where subcultural knowledge regarding use and access to the drugs is growing – shows the value of collective action as a groundswell for cultural change.

Indeed, community knowledge-building and sharing, developed socially and through collective practices and infrastructures, provides a vision of bodily support, possibility, and transformation, proposing other ways of embodied being, or even of collective health. In Preciado's frame, it describes the 'transformation of the body of the multitude into an open living political archive: the common *somathéque*', situating the ensouled bodymind amid open-source gender codes.[59] Given the particular forms of pathologising medical scrutiny that trans and non-binary people face, it is unsurprising that our DIY/DIT practices face public disdain outside of our communities – especially so from psychiatrists who otherwise have power over our access to healthcare. Trans and non-binary people will continue to need to share our skills and knowledge, to upskill, to develop medical skills within our communities, and to build autonomous infrastructure for the purposes of harm reduction. While, following Gleeson and Hoad who describe the free sharing of 'collective knowledge and experience' regarding gender transition and trans-affirmative healthcare as 'seeds' of a potentially 'emancipated practice',[60] the question is perhaps how self-medding gets transformed from a marginalised practice into an emancipatory one. Emancipation entails the reduction of harm in the realm of medical safety in order to thrive – we discuss the framework of Liberatory Harm Reduction at the end of this chapter.

Private healthcare is accessible for some by sourcing financial aid from within a marginalised community that is often – but by no means always – financially precarious.[61] While this might take care of an individual's pressing needs, it underlines how financial and social inequalities push people deeper into unfair systems of distribution. Such resourcing no doubt also contains racial and class separations, and may mean that *sometimes* limited financial resources are being shared between people who have little; however, it's worth remembering that financial redistribution is an important element of the forms of social transformation that will counter the logics of racial capitalist accumulation, separability and enforced scarcity. Under the fiscal logics of scarcity and organised abandonment, private providers may stand ready to exploit our needs, as is the status quo in most places where healthcare operates for profit;[62] although, what is gained through these grammars of extraction is our health. Redistribution of both finances and skills are political actions we can undertake, towards harm reduction and making trans life more liveable – these are means of countering the logics of accumulation, separability and scarcity. However, these are practices whereby the collectives we are involved with may have to reach outside of their comfort zones.

NO BROWN PUSSIES

A personal story that speaks to a political situation.[63] I (Nat) start the year 2019 on a precipice of claiming agency over my bodymind. At the same time and place, a friend and I are attending appointments for surgical consultations. The appointments are at a private hospital that the NHS contracts for this particular surgery – at this time, there is one place, one surgeon, and healthcare team that we have access to through the NHS route where we live (Scotland).[64] At this point in my interrelation with gender-affirming healthcare, it's the *third* time I've been through the GIC system to get to the point of a successful referral for gender-affirming surgery,[65] having first been referred to a GIC in 2007 only to be denied healthcare and discharged a couple of years later. As radical trans healthcare activists, we've taken to describing the people involved in the ongoing psychiatrisation of trans-specific healthcare in the UK the Gender Identity Cops (or 'gender cops' for short). This description emerges primarily because psychiatrists, who retain the top jobs at GICs and ultimately have power over access to healthcare through a GIC, remain invested in socially conservative gender norms. The clinic understands transsexuality through a Eurocentric conception of gender as primarily based on a sex/gender binary, with intersex and non-binary people making up knowable exceptions in the view of more progressive doctors. The clinic remains invested in judging the proceedings of medical transitions (from M to F, or F to M), gender expressions (men look and dress one way, women look and dress that way, non-binary people are literally up for debate) and that 'patients' are 'stable' within socially conservative forms of life (monogamy, heteronormativity, stable employment, the family, etc.).

As per the GIC, my friend has tipped me off to expect being patronised by the 'gender team' at this private healthcare provider too. A group of nurses (all older, white, and cisgender) speak to us – a group of trans women and trans femmes from different age groups, including another person I've met at an activist meeting – about practicalities regarding surgery. What is required of us prior to surgery, what to expect while in hospital, and how the recovery period will go. This includes what to pack for a week in hospital, surgical options, recovery and refraining from physical activity, and hygiene. Some of this is organisational, some of it detail, and some of it strangely alienating: we're spoken to in a matter that assumes one has little experience of any of these things including personal hygiene; and in a highlight of cisnormativity, we're advised to expect post-op bleeding that will be 'like your first period'.

We're holding our tongues, given our experiences of having the healthcare we need gate-kept from us; given the number of hoops we have jumped through and appointments with psychiatrists to get to this stage. The medical – or biopolitical – power that is held over trans bodies is real and material: it has an influence on the physical condition of our bodyminds. It can also be wielded in a seriously harmful and sometimes murderous, necropolitical manner through denying the healthcare we need – causing distress, serious harm, and devastating psychological impacts.

The confrontation with transmisogynist and cis-normative attitudes towards trans women, trans femmes, and non-binary people pursuing treatments remains a standard affair in the GIC system and private sector contractors, given its conservative, Eurocentric conceptions of gender norms and transsexuality. To treat trans women, femmes and non-binary people in a demeaning manner around something that has major life stakes for us, forces us in line with conservative gender norms in order to access surgeries and treatments. Here, the cisnormativity manifests in the assumptions that only women – that is cisgender women – menstruate (there are trans and non-binary people who menstruate); that it's an 'essential' part of 'womanhood' (there are cisgender women who don't menstruate); and it suggests that trans women understand our bodies in practice through a cis-normative lens.

The practice of these norms also assumes that our ensouled bodyminds – and what we do and wish to do with them – fit into white, primarily hetero and cis-normative ideas of sexuality and gender. Trans and non-binary people face these latter assumptions commonly in everyday life, but in the clinic I face them firstly in the denial of healthcare to my brown queer trans femme bodymind, and then in the subjection of my bodymind to its healthcare regime.

Back at the appointment, the gender team nurses discuss possible surgical options, also speaking about the visual ('cosmetic') results for those of us who signed up to get new pussies. Indeed, cisgender women and trans women (and some non-binary people) do go through similar medical procedures that entail redesigning vulvas (labiaplasty) and remaking vaginas (vaginoplasty). The discussion of cosmetic results includes flicking through what is colloquially described as 'The Big Book of [Neo-]Vulvas', illustrated with surgical results, showing vulvas at various stages of healing. Not all vulvas look the same, and each image in the book has its own dynamic. However, one thing remains consistent in its visual domain: they all belong to bodies that would be racialised as white.

Putting aside that skin colour includes the skin of one's genitals, I'm initially surprised that the book doesn't speak to the embodiment of (trans) people of colour, although as far as I'm aware I'm the only woman of colour in the room.

In the weeks following the appointment – one that was tied up with high stakes regarding invasive procedures – I started to count how many Black and Brown trans people I'd encountered over the years in the waiting rooms of the clinics, dating back to the mid-2000s (low single figures, and they really do make you wait in there); and how few close Brown and Black trans friends had received the healthcare they desired from the GIC. Most trans people of colour I could think of had pursued private healthcare for even the basics – Hormone Replacement Therapy, topical treatments such as hair removal, alongside surgeries too, myself included. I remember having to pay for private healthcare, out of my student loan, in my early 20s, which quickly lapsed into having no specialist healthcare when I could no longer afford private treatment, having graduated into unemployment. I remembered a story of another desi trans person, who was fighting delays in receiving treatment from the GIC, because the GIC didn't understand the cultural codes of gender around their name. I reflect on the history of racism in healthcare; the contemporary and past struggles of migrants to get the healthcare they/we need, including recently introduced charges and passport checks at the point of access, or due to the horrors of immigration detention and incarceration.

In telling this story,[66] we want to emphasise how whiteness undergirds both the construction of who the 'patient' is when it comes to gender-affirming healthcare and/or healthcare in Europe more broadly, and who make up the embodied ideal subjects of trans epistemologies in psychiatry, but also in our own understandings of transness. The gender binary itself is one of the technologies of coloniality, an imposition forming part of projects of empire – used to dispossess Indigenous peoples and their lands, while gender was also reserved for the domain subject of the 'human' (white people).[67] As C. Riley Snorton discusses, gynaecology as a science has roots in the exploitation of the bodies of enslaved Black women in the nineteenth century.[68] Aren Aizura reminds us that the psychiatric conceptualisation of transsexuality was constructed through whiteness; and also how transness has repeatedly relied on orientalising metaphors of travel.[69] Prominent narratives around medical gender transition in the UK – even the reflexive and politicised ones – have been primarily authored by white trans people.[70] If what it means to shift between or away from the poles of the colonial gender binary is also encoded in and through white bodyminds, the space for Black, Indigenous, and other trans people of colour to articulate ourselves to medical practitioners through global majority cultural understandings (or through diasporic ones) of gender and transness narrows – shrinking the likelihood of receiving healthcare that meets our needs. We find ourselves having to translate our embodied understandings into the bifurcations of Western medicine (including a body/mind split, of physical and mental health), or of understanding ourselves through them too.

ON RACIAL INFRASTRUCTURES IN HEALTHCARE

To speak of healthcare – and specifically the NHS – as a racial infrastructure is to highlight that the genesis and functioning of this health service is inextricable from the dynamics of racial capitalism. By infrastructure, we mean the material infrastructure of a system or provision, that is the labour and capital – the workers, the resources, the equipment, medicines, buildings, and of course the money – that are oriented towards the support of a service. In the case of a health service, we're speaking of a system designed to support living through infirmity and sickness, to assist disability and debility, to enable reproduction and life, often in the time of birth or amid prospects of death. It is an infrastructure designed to assist social reproduction, such that we can continue to live and often to work, to be productive individuals within a national economy. In the case of the NHS, this service was historically proposed to be a social healthcare system, paid for via taxation and free at the point of access. In recent years, however, the introduction of charges for prescriptions in England, or missed appointments, and moreover the forms of insurance charged to migrants, have functioned as a contradiction to this ethos. The public is consistently reminded – by politicians and bureaucracy – that the NHS costs the public purse, and that 'wasting' time entails wasting money under a rubric of the efficient use of resources; during the COVID-19 pandemic, we were instructed by the government to 'Protect the NHS' – although this stopped neither mass death nor the outsourcing of further NHS resources developed to manage the pandemic, which themselves had mixed results.[71]

In recent years, we've been reminded by political commentators that the capital on which the NHS was founded, in the late 1940s after World War II, was inextricable from the project of the British Empire.[72] This was the time of formal decolonisation, where those of us who had been colonised by the British fought the state for freedom and independence, giving rise to independent nation-states amidst major unrest, violence, and famine.[73] Historically, from the Windrush Generation, and to the present – the NHS has depended upon migrant workers in order to function, across the levels ranging between doctors, nurses, and cleaners. As noted in 2021 by the British Medical Association (BMA), 'the UK has always recruited directly from the colonies and former colonies to fill short-staffed positions in the NHS'. Migrant workers from the Caribbean, South Asia, and East Asia have been essential to the operations of the NHS from its outset; the health service has been able to source this labour through the relations and legacies of the British Commonwealth. The BMA underlines that, compared to other organisations in the UK, the NHS is unique in that its workforce is 'significantly more racially diverse than the general UK population'.[74]

The BMA identify that the overrepresentation of ethnic minorities across lower-paid roles in the NHS – who meanwhile have more 'negative experience and lower confidence in organisations' – is indicative of structural racism within the organisation.[75] Structural racism is also evident in the study of medicine – from pass rates to experiences of bullying – and in career progression and opportunities once qualifying. A recent series of texts on racism, xenophobia, discrimination, and health in *The Lancet* discuss how, in the field of health, 'systemic racism is instilled through professional training and education, with the conditioning and learning of whiteness (and maleness) as the norm'.[76] The authors emphasise that this is undergirded by colonial logics that established social hierarchies on race and indigeneity, gender and language.[77] Structural racism is, of course, also fed further by economic shifts that compound working conditions and experiences in health services – the underfunding of the NHS leading to an intensification of workloads, with record numbers of NHS staff leaving the service in 2022 (for a variety of reasons, including work-life balance and retirement, but in a climate of concern for the stress on GPs in particular).[78]

In a time where the political claim that Black Lives Matter has been heard across the world, we question how health infrastructures are working for Black people, Indigenous people, and people of colour, and migrants more broadly. We know that both the NHS user charges introduced in recent years for non-UK citizens, alongside the functioning of the Hostile Environment within the health service, will likely affirm a racialised economy of health and care in the UK. Specifically identifying the discrepancies in treatment between Black trans and non-binary people, trans people of colour, and white trans people in the UK GIC system requires further research. However, in pointing towards dynamics of racism within provisions for gender-affirmative/trans-specific healthcare, including the use of Eurocentric conceptions of trans and non-binary (which, in the case of these framings affecting the work of the Gender Clinic, could also be studied further), we hope to make space to develop these dialogues further among trans, non-binary, and non-trans people. In the spirit of a transfeminist ethics, there is work we can do among ourselves to challenge these dynamics – to centre or create space for Black, South Asian, East Asian, and Indigenous people, and perspectives within healthcare activism; to provide space for expansive conceptions of health that may challenge Western assumptions; to recognise how whiteness can and does play into our interactions with healthcare providers, down to the languages and grammars of gender and transness we use to gain leverage and power through our bodies, especially when seeking treatment from medical professionals and psychiatrists. That the imaginary of the trans movement, shifting between rights and provisions, has to work to undo its racial limits when it comes to building or proposing alternatives to infrastructures for living. Within trans organising, we need to ensure that our practices within collectives and communities take into account how racism and xenophobia affect our access to trans-specific and broader healthcare;[79] and in addition, work to address differentials and separation/separability within our worlds and social ecologies; creating space to have conversations connecting our experiences and their underlying dynamics.

LIBERATORY HARM REDUCTION:
A PROPOSAL TO RETHINK AUTONOMY

To think through strategies to deal with the dire state of trans healthcare, we will look at Shira Hassan's work on Liberatory Harm Reduction. While Hassan's work emerges from the social dynamics of substance use, there are insights that are very helpful for a reconceptualisation of the ethics surrounding trans health care. This is in part because Hassan thinks through a strong abolitionist framework and is working from a deep understanding of the violence within institutions and institutionalised violence.

Let's start with a particularly devastating insight from Sarah Daoud:

> One easy way to know for sure that corporate nonprofits aren't practicing Liberatory Harm Reduction: they're the same ones doling out punishments that keep people unsafe and unwell, that force you into compliance over self-determination [...] forcibly medicating you or sterilizing you and on and on and on. They're supposed to be where you get help, but often they're actually sites of violence. *It creates a culture where young folks are afraid to ask for help, because help usually comes with harm and control.*[80]

While we will talk about self-determination later, here let's focus on the problem that asking for 'help usually comes with harm and control'.

The moment people get to choose their own directions in life, a sense of agency enables the imagination of other worlds. One is not, in these moments, constrained by the categories of perception that others use to impose limits on them.[81] However, as we have discussed in the last chapter, the ruse of institutions is that they only offer choices of pre-existing pathways in the institution. Sarah Daoud concludes 'these systems seek to control us, punish us for being "defiant", and then toss us out when we can't function as they demand'.[82] When engaging medical institutions – and here we differ from some of the staging of Hassan's discussion – it seems unlikely that we would be able to 'choose' our way out of the mess of violence, condescension, and bad care. There is something else we need, something that stretches beyond individualised agency, to tackle the limiting approaches of institutions.

The four pillars of medical ethics are benevolence, no maleficence, autonomy, and (informed) consent. This sounds great. However, the forced sterilisations of trans people in Europe were carried out under the banner of these four pillars.[83] Pathologisation of trans people, punishment culture, and the endemic condescension of clinicians can all be made to fit into these approaches. This is in part because they are quite abstract, and in part because medical institutions are structured very hierarchically. Informed consent in a hierarchical and specialised environment can amount to little more than giving doctors permission to do what they think is necessary when the pathology is structured around social devaluation, such as trans. In specialised care, informed consent should mean that people understand what will happen, what the other options are, and what their expectations are following medical intervention. However, in trans care informed consent has often meant compliance with the clinician's pathology, rather than agency about what one actually wants. In contrast to formal medical ethics, the Liberatory Harm Reduction framework starts from the user and their space for agency in limiting conditions (bodily/mentally, socially, structurally, and institutionally) and stretches that out into an abolitionist approach. This last step enables extending from individualised people, who have to make their 'own' choices, to collectives supporting the navigation of supportive and hostile systems.

Liberatory Harm Reduction is a strategy for organising for survival and building collectives emerging from Black and Brown trans people, such as Marsha P. Johnson, Sylvia Rivera, and Miss Major Griffin-Gracy. Tourmaline considers it a gift, and as such it should be accepted with grace and treated with respect. It is a strategy for action against disposability.[84] To cite a part of the definition:

> Liberatory Harm Reduction is a philosophy [...] that teach[es] us to accompany each other as we transform the root causes of harm in our lives. We put our values into action using real-life strategies to reduce the negative health, legal and social consequences that result from criminalised and stigmatised life-experiences [...] Liberatory Harm Reductionists support each other and our communities without judgement or stigma or coercion, and we do not force others to change [...] Liberatory Harm Reduction is true self-determination and total body autonomy.[85]

This way of seeing helps us to imagine and practice ways of supporting each other through transformation, and how to work against stigma without coercion. At times trans people in Europe call for 'informed consent', but here we want to emphasise that Liberatory Harm Reduction offers better strategies to think through our engagement with medical institutions. It emerges from abolitionist frameworks and does not, ultimately, see the institution as the saviour that needs to be made to include trans folk. We might need the medical institution as a service provider and resource distributor, but once we are in contact with them as users, it is key to emphasise harm reduction – and most of all: approaching trans health care as a *body-loving practice*. Reading those words in Hassan's description of SEXXY – a young people's needle exchange programme in Chicago – left me, Mijke, thunderstruck.[86] It framed in a flash how body-hating the treatment at the VU Gender Clinic in Amsterdam had been. This body-hating emerges in part from the emphasis in medical circles that only by adapting the body to the pathologised mind will allow a transgender healing of sorts. In the 1990s and 2000s, there was a lot of talk amongst trans people about hating their own bodies – the 'born in the wrong body' trope was alive and kicking. From my background as a dancer, this was not my story, but it was hard to escape its pressure, isolated in an environment that holds no love for who (body and mind) you are. For starters, one had to convince the psychologists that one was 'depressed' but only because of transness, not for any other reason. So, one had to self-pathologise and display sadness to access medication. The endocrinologists, minus one, were indifferent, and to this day I am aware of how a lighter dose of testosterone suppressor might have changed my entire perception of how to navigate my time at the clinic. The dose they prescribed, as was then standard, was high and numbed an entire section of our body-minds. This was done 'because we wanted it', without there being a conversation about whether we wanted a numb pelvis. Instead, if one questioned something, one was threatened with being pushed out of the programme. Harm and control indeed. How differently will a clinic look if it centres on body-loving practices? This thought returns us lovingly to Travis Alabanza's reminder that 'we do this for us, baby' – the musings that 'baby' is a term of endearment, (sometimes) a reminder of our youth, and that 'like a baby, I could start again, and mould and shift – learn to talk again, if I must'.[87] Seriously, we have only one bodymind and we get to do everything with ourselves: be that self-medding, substance use, sex, work, and play, etc. It is this bodily being that we better surround with care as love, rather than with clinical approaches based on rejecting ourselves, which is yet another normative strategy for harming trans people.

In light of this discussion, another leading political aim and slogan that could use further reflection is *full bodily autonomy*. Our hesitation with this idea arises from philosophical, ethical, and strategic angles. We affirm the idea that when a decision comes close to one's bodymind, is about what happens to oneself, or even which actions to take, there needs to be a sense of agency and the possibility of being responsible for oneself.[88] This is what undergirds twenty-first-century political demands for autonomy, including for abortion rights. However, an emphasis on personal choice – which is where radical and liberal approaches meet – within a neoliberal environment emphasises empowering *the individual*. As we discussed in Chapter 3, when one pits the individual against the institution, the individual loses. It is a real question of how much autonomy can rescue oneself in a Hostile Environment. It also puts a huge demand on people to make it through institutions by their own wits, rather than supported by a collective; to navigate institutions is a middle-class asset, and some people have not been trained in this skill.

The idea of autonomy emerges in modern times from Immanuel Kant, who took it out of a reading of Machiavelli. Machiavelli used the idea of autonomy literally to mean 'giving oneself the law' in the context of the self-rule of city-states. Kant took this idea and turned it inward – for Kant it made sense to imagine that a rational society would be governed through a universal morality, where everybody behaves as a lawgiver, with (imaginary) laws that would count for everyone.[89] Kant individualises autonomy, rather than seeing it as collective. Kant's project assumed everybody thinks in the same way (universal rationality), which is why this individualisation of choice would not dissolve into chaos or confrontation. This lineage is why autonomy is problematic from a philosophical angle: it assumes we think as law-givers, and that we make our choices by ourselves (even though Kant assumed a non-relational, but rational collectivity running in the background). However, this idea of individual choice might harm us (but not worse than having someone else impose their pathologies upon us).

From the angle of ethics, the appeal of Liberatory Harm Reduction lies in its emphasis on *accompanying each other*, to *support each other and our communities*, and doing so without *judgement, stigma or coercion*. This can be summarised in the phrase *we do not force others to change*. This emphasis offers a deep ethics, it is relational, collective, and is aware of the space people need to step up to transformation. Its power is in the collective, not in the choices of the individual self. Otherwise, the empowered middle class with their individual choices would produce the best outcome. But it is clear why they don't: this approach lacks collective responsibility, the absence of judgement and involves coercion, and often – as middle managers – it forces others to change. What they do have aplenty is individual choice, almost as Kant meant it to be – choice that is empowered by institutions. In environments with a strong middle-class conceptual grounding, such as those populated by people who went through Further or Higher Education, emphasising autonomy might be a strategic way to get people into collective work. However, when we look at the deep ethics in Liberatory Harm Reduction, what makes it radical, transformative, and loving is that it emphasises collectivity without coercion. And that is where its real strength lies: it entails collectivity that everyone is open to aligning with, as long as they leave coercion behind.

The strategic part flows from here. First, we can be hesitant to accept that one of the key modernist philosophical tools will lead to liberation, however seductive it is. Second, if institutions coerce under the heading of individual choice, making one responsible for choices made under coercion – such as with the forced sterilisation of trans people in Europe, which happened under the heading of autonomy – what we might need is to bring the collective into the environment. Sarah Daoud reminds us of this:

> Liability laws and other bureaucracy make honoring what people want to do with their bodies nearly impossible [...] So, we're given public health harm reduction, and told it's the same thing. That it's good enough. It's like what they say in cooking shows – if you can't make your own, store bought is fine. But most of the time, state sanctioned harm reduction isn't fine. It's the site of harm.[90]

Individualised choice within the institution cannot function as harm reduction, because of the tension between individual choice, and how choice emerges from collective living. Choice in institutions follows delimited routes, which are preserved through punishment or the threat of exclusion.

We are not trying to give a one-size-fits-all solution. What is at stake for us is to liberate thinking from the trap of individualised choices within institutions. Harm reduction in medical settings allows a user-driven slow experiment, contra the context of harm. While the effects and side-effects of HRT are well known for non-trans people and well discussed within trans communities – although seemingly under-researched in regard to trans people in medical literature – user-driven variations with medical support allow for a huge experimental field to adjust the pharmaceutical disinterest in gender-specific medication. Edinburgh Action for Trans Health called for this approach in 2017; its traces are also in Preciado's *Testo Junkie*.[91] If such an experiment is body-loving, user-directed, and collective, it enables adjusting some of the hierarchies present in medical settings. It is one step in moving towards collective spaces without having to give up our sense of agency. Medical settings can be opened up to sociality and lead to imagining other worlds.

The hierarchy of institutions seemingly homogenises users, because people are seen as needing to fit into an existing white European frame. Mariame Kaba offers that

> what stuck with me through the years is a resistance to the idea that 'difference is determinative'. Just because I come from a different place than somebody else does not mean that we cannot figure out ways to work together, or that we cannot contribute in ways that allow us to bring our unique selves to the process.[92]

Institutions do not often make time for this, and medical institutions approach people as patients who need to be dealt with individually. In the case of trans, this is a peculiar approach, because as we have proposed throughout this book, *trans is a relational process*. This does not mean that we propose 'group diagnosis', but that we engender a space where healthcare providers actually support, in a functional and affirmative way, a social process. This needs to replace the top-down testing of people to see if they fit within a pathology, which from the outset treats people with suspicion, rather than care, as has been the practice of the Gender Clinic historically.

The call to depathologise trans is part of the call to end this suspicion and to restore agency. It is a call to end hierarchical approaches that trap people in violent structures set up to fail those who are struggling. In that sense, to ask for care in a vulnerable moment and be met by what Daoud analyses as 'harm and control', is to be feminised – to let the trans person know the impact of (yet another) demoted social status. The waiting lists, the arrogance of medical staff, the judgemental and invasive questions, the indifference of endocrinologists, and the unavailability of surgeons are all part of an atmosphere of violence that lets trans people know they are not a priority. As we discussed above, waiting times and violence experienced in medical space are a source of trauma in themselves – this trauma reinforces the pathologisation of trans as a category, and it disrupts relationality and potentiality. Waiting times and disruptions to the lives of trans people lead some of us to lag behind our peers, creating disadvantages in our lives, further adding to stigma in a neoliberal regime that emphasises individual responsibility. This underlines how hierarchies benefit from ways in which people are held back (for instance, in workplaces, any excuse not to advance people will be taken, to ensure the space at the top is not overcrowded). Remember: who guards something owns it – and healthcare, workplaces, education, and other resources are all part of that scarcity-property mindset. Abolishing the policing of trans in medical settings will make space for engendering our bodyminds and our lives.

SOLIDARITY ACROSS HEALTHCARE STRUGGLES

Through building wider solidarity among feminist healthcare struggles, and sharing and developing collective practices between these struggles, we grow and politicise our understanding of experiences that are typically individualised. (Consciousness-raising, as this has been known since the 1970s.) Feminist healthcare struggles are a key node of interdependency and care: sharing maps of well-trodden pathways, replete with attendant challenges and difficulties, helps to situate an individual within a wider context, to understand the embodied politics of one's experience, and to assemble shared social and collective means of overcoming difficulties. Feminist coalitions across movements against femicide, transfemicide, and domestic violence, and for Black liberation, reproductive justice, and disability justice, have dozens of logical interconnections. Trans, non-binary, and queer analytics produce clear points of convergence, provided these movements can eclipse any latent transphobia and (trans)misogyny. Such coalitional feminist collectives are active across the globe, from Brazil and Mexico to the US and UK. For instance, in the Summer of 2020, Black Lives Matter demonstrations focused on Black transfemicides in the US, as Black trans women organisers rallied tens of thousands of people into the streets of Brooklyn and London highlighting the deaths of Layleen Polanco and Tony McDade in police custody, and the deaths of Rem'mie Fells, Riah Milton and Naomi Hersi. In spite of a backlash against abortion rights, feminists have secured victories through coalitional organising, such as in Argentina.[93] In these struggles for reproductive rights, trans people have been central, such as the Frente Trans Masculin. The dire state of trans healthcare, and anti-trans attacks on trans healthcare provisions, have repoliticised gender-affirming care as an issue. However, the healthcare needs of trans people reach well beyond the provisions of the Gender Clinic.

There are multiple issues through which coalitional struggles around healthcare, across non-trans, non-binary, and trans people, can be forged. Indeed, the particularity with which trans-specific healthcare is approached smooths access to effective and accessible healthcare for everyone. The exceptionalisation of trans people in research – when there is, for instance, seemingly limited research on trans people and long-term HRT use – works to isolate us from knowledge. Nonetheless, trans knowledges align with other approaches to epistemic injustice that emphasise the need to involve marginalised subjects under study in all aspects of research (from design and ethics to authorship). HRT is a common intervention in bodily processes for many of us – people who take HRT for menopausal symptoms may not be aware that they share the same medication as trans people. When we compare notes across supposed differences, it allows for knowledge exchange between circles that builds up over decades. HRT shortages in the UK post-Brexit – in a context where the public is impelled by politicians to feel 'grateful' for the NHS, while it has been chronically underfunded by Conservative and Labour Governments – affect all users, as do the limited options of HRT medications available. Advocacy for more options, a wider range of medications, and the licensing of medications that are regularly used in other countries is important.

Similarly, reproductive rights issues are often framed through cis-normative language, which can make them appear separate to trans healthcare struggles – however, trans people do also require to access abortions.[94] Given that right-wing politicians endeavour to curtail abortion access in general, the struggle for better abortion access is a shared struggle; furthermore, we are deeply in need of clinics that centre issues of race in reproductive care.[95] Trans and non-binary struggles for reproductive justice can work to undo other norms in accessing assistive technologies and natal care.[96] The separation of struggles makes our struggles harder; care is a litmus test of how stark social hierarchies in our world impact our bodies and lives directly.

Making a collective world is also about resources: the politics of care is about prioritising, nurturing, and nourishing embodied life – with labour and with time. We do this as a practice of challenging racial and gendered separability. Healthcare is the site where social struggles meet because it centres on how our bodies meet the world. In that sense healthcare struggles are about more than healthcare – they are about creating a world where we can trust each other with our lives.

5

Abolitionist transfeminist futures

Solidarity, generosity and love

Surely there must be another way out? [...] What is it we're living for?

— Letta Mbulu, 'What's Wrong With Groovin'

Underneath all the thundering there's magic and if there's a better way to live, I've gotta have it.

— Kneecap, 'Better Way to Live'

SKILLS FOR SHARED FUTURES

The groundwork of transformation falls upon all of us who want to be in solidarity with existences that are not tied to the circumstances of birth (gender, class, race, caste, ability). Such groundwork emerges from everyday solidarity that diminishes harm. We believe that the shaping of transfeminist futures, which are abolitionist, collective, and intermesh with Black feminist futures and that gather those who Saidiya Hartman would describe as wayward – engaged in surviving and living otherwise[1] – is essential to the liberation and survival of all of us. These are futures grounded in refusing disposability and separability. The emergence of trans liberation depends on form, rather than content. In other words, it depends on *how* we get together, our practices, worlding, and grassroots organising shape ways to enable the 'freedoms' of our lives and our ensouled bodyminds.[2] The fabrication and intermeshing of the futures we actually wish to live is a collective task, one whose sustenance requires our reflection and engagement. In Lola Olufemi's words, '[n]ot *otherwise* as in, the political horizon awaits; *otherwise* as in, a firm embrace of the unknowable'.[3]

By orienting our time, skills and other resources towards each other, the future can emerge as our collective dreams as they unfold. In the words of the Atelier Manifesto, it entails 'return[ing] the creative force into dreams of defiance and resistance, justice and freedom, happiness and kindness, friendship and wonderment' – into our practices of living and entanglement with each other.[4] Part of our argument has been that it is not content but form that allows the possibility of a radical departure of norms. We discussed modes of relation to make new lives through care in Chapter 2. On a larger scale, we questioned how solidarity can take shape *vis-à-vis* the demands of institutions in Chapters 3 and 4. Transfeminism, which is our formulation of *how* we get together, proposes alternative practices to resist the structures that keep us isolated and separated, by addressing how we remain ensnared in these structures. In this sense, we have offered a departure from recognition-based accounts, and accounts that centre homogenous groups – such accounts often rest on positionality, how one is socially located.[5] Instead, we have theorised collectivity through ethics, which describes the direction that I, or we, try to move in. These directions are not always visible and can be understood as the work that needs to be done to bloom new futures in the present. We expect that this work dissolves positionalities that took shape under racist, sexist, and capitalist regimes, without giving up on the knowledges that histories of oppression offer. This importantly includes the need to share knowledge, histories, and practices across generations.

The ethics we propose seeks shared forms that emerge from within a strongly pluriversal world.[6] We understand the pluriverse as the 'reimagining and reconstructing of local worlds' in connection to each other without a dominating single epistemology or politics.[7] Thinking through pluriversal forms means that we are committed to a horizontal approach, to curb one form overshadowing other forms – i.e. in contrast to the hierarchical approaches that institutions, borders, and states enforce. In queer circles (both academic and collective), we feel that leaning on indeterminacy, which we know from queer theory since the 1990s,[8] has blocked speaking about forms we make in practice. The connections, priorities, and ways of relating in the spaces in which we bring our (ensouled) bodyminds together and share our lives, constitute a trans ethics. Even when resistance does not start with radical forms, part of the struggle is to open spaces and ourselves more and extend towards different futures. Anne-Marie Quinn, in conversation with other former Political Prisoners from Armagh Gaol, reflects that 'People [in Northern Ireland] have learnt a lot about conflict resolution and transformation and transition from conflict. Any country that ever had a victory, an all-out overnight victory, it doesn't last long. So, the idea of constant negotiating and trying to find a way forward is really what we need.'[9] Quinn underlines that the work political agents are doing in the present is slow because it doesn't focus on quick wins, but on finding ways forward together, addressing friction, as we discuss below, as a way to make new futures.

In the present moment of climate crisis, necrocapitalistic fatalism, global corporate power, continuous war, mass incarceration, and in the face of despair, our envisioning and its activation is a strength. Coming together calls for both distributing our skills and upskilling and relying on each other, in and beyond trans and queer movements. Furthermore, we address the dynamics undergirding transphobia within feminist movements. We analyse and reflect on these dynamics through an abolitionist framework – that refuses a politics of innocence – in order to underline the responsibility of all feminists to collectively reckon with our capacity to decry and also harm each other. It demands that we approach each other with care, curiosity, and generosity, practising gratitude for what we make between us. In this last chapter, we look at skills as ways to face our own participation in harm, making solidarity, as ways to love, and nurture joy. We look at this transfeminist ethics as a way to discuss how we can emerge in new futures, collectively and without isolating ourselves.

AN ETHICS OF GENEROSITY

Movement work provides a clear counterpoint to the logics of extraction, and contractual and exchanged-based relations. It carries within it both the promise and practice of non-exploitative living, provided movements and those of us who make them practice an openness to (forms of) life, and to change. Generosity in our approaches, we propose here, is key to this. Movement work draws on the skills of friendship.[10] Friendship does not consist of an offer of emotional labour, but it is rather a form of generosity within relations where labour cannot reach. Therefore, we consider generosity as a foundation for living and openness to life, which is material, emotional, intellectual, and practical. The main element is that a generous approach is founded on trust in others.[11] As a modality of care, generosity as a shared practice enhances the vibrant character of collectives. It interrupts contractual foci and legalistic approaches because it cannot be codified in the law. Generosity as a disposition affords space to bodies, communities, and forms of life, and relies on openness and solidarity as part of the grain of attitudes and actions. Rather than setting the terms of the engagement, like the law or contracts, such an attitude invites imagination and curiosity.

In the previous chapters we argued for grounding sociality in complicity, to reshape our entanglements in participation and resistance, and to depart from an entrenched dichotomy of social structure versus experience. We discussed how complicity shifts perpetrator–victim narratives that make passivity synonymous with disempowered people. Here, we add to this the idea that solidarity offers an ethics whereby participation in transfeminist struggles aims for the total liberation of everyone, while leaving the direction of the struggle open and avoiding being overtly prescriptive.[12] We can engage in struggles and shared resistance in the present, while our orientation to the future can remain open to what we will collectively forge, play, and dream together. Openness requires you to practice things you might be bad at (perhaps at first, perhaps forever) and forgive yourself (and others) for it. It suggests experimentation. In this sense, generosity is playful as María Lugones emphasises, opening us towards logics that are not one's own; indeed we might call it anarchic – without hierarchical ordering – with the aid of Marquis Bey.[13] To be open entails softening one's perspective and releasing certainties.

Combined with an embrace of complicity, generosity requires putting oneself at stake in the struggle for transformation and, also, for our worlds in their beauty. It emerges through the dynamics and actions required to show our appreciation for people, collectives, flora and fauna in our movements and worlds. And yet, generosity is not only celebratory. Generous attention to the patterns in which life unfolds also opens space for mourning: for the vibrations of those that we lost, of what we have lost, and of the knowledge and skills of *how* to do things that might still be out of reach. We are participants in the struggle for liberation, rather than disembedded observers. Together, we can break enclosures, and return everything to everyone.

Yet a key problem under the conditions of patriarchal racial capitalism is that femininity may be read to represent opportunity, ease, scope to control and dominate, flexibility, sexualisation, and a provision of free labour and care (with or without consent) – all of which can be exploited, as we discussed in Chapter 2. However, it's in collectives, communities, and movements that the exploitation of generosity will sting in a different manner. We might say that to 'take advantage' of generosity – rather than practice relations of mutuality – is to move through collective/communal/transformative spaces in a bourgeois manner. This bourgeois manner is a middle-class entitlement that remains grounded in extractivism and exploitation, and that relies on the care and invisibilised labour of others.[14] In the expectations placed upon femmes to care for others, care can come to feel laborious and extractive; the love that is practised may not be reciprocated in kind, and the work may be more easily made invisible or forgotten by the movement.[15] A willingness to share is a point that soft patriarchy will exploit.[16] Drawing on circumstances to ask for a surrender of our needs, desires, and activities, usually under the guise of reasonability, has been a hallmark of paternalist approaches.[17]

Nonetheless, we are interdependent – and our worlds do not exist without each other.[18] The willingness to share and make space is the strong point of feminist approaches. We want to offer and act in the world with generosity towards those we build worlds with, and those we wish or intend to join us; if generosity is mutual, its touch will be met when we ask for it, and sometimes offered because a need is noticed. The possibility of exploitation should never support the argument to stop a practice of generosity, but generosity does at times require the willingness to create friction within collectives. Such attempts at exploitation are inevitable – yet raising and challenging exploitation is not. Responding to the friction with refusal is an opportunity to learn its sources, and to teach how to change through refusal.[19] Simultaneously, affective clues that we might have used to navigate *hostile* spaces, including a sense of victimhood or hurt innocence when being closed out of institutions, are often not constructive for approaching collective spaces. A sense of responsibility and generosity might interrupt these intuitions.

SOLIDARITY, CLOUDBUSTING, AND FACING THE MESS

Solidarity remains the key dynamic of the social world (despite and in spite of the neoliberal end of history), affirming the transformative power that we can manifest together. In this chapter, we reflect on practices of transfeminist solidarity within wider feminist collective organising – its successes, problems, and ways to work through these. It returns us, again, to consider how we work across and through difference, and what we learn together through it.

The dynamics of marginalisation and fetishisation of trans femmes and women are interrelated, both socially and sexually. Fetishisation, here, is partly about sexual objectification, but also about a reduction of people to a categorical identity – that by 'fact' of being a trans woman, one emerges as an overdetermined set of character-types, behaviours, experience, and embodiment, to be understood as such for the sake of inclusion. At the same time, we find ourselves navigating, countering, reflecting, and internalising the cultural climate of anti-trans hostility, including in our everyday practices. The climate, here, may be best understood in the manner that Christina Sharpe articulates the climate of anti-Blackness as 'the weather', an all-encompassing surrounding in which we live, work, and organise.[20] This is not to say that the climate of anti-transness is the same as the climate of anti-Blackness – such climates are co-constitutive of each other, as we learn in the work of C. Riley Snorton and Marquis Bey.[21] But it is to suggest that the climates of anti-Blackness, anti-transness – and of racism, xenophobia, and ableism more broadly – are not just structural, institutional, or produced by forces seemingly external to our social lives and practices. The climate is the socialities and affective economies we are situated within, and can be complicit in reproducing them and actively dismantling them. We may be a part of it, and (set) apart from it. In the context of the laws and technologies of separability, we adopt practices of cloudbusting in our everyday lives which may be as simple as showing up when we've been taught to stay away; to reflecting upon and challenging embodied responses which may have been affected by these climates of hate. You could say that one gets 'conditioned' into reproducing these climates, but that suggests a factual, enduring state of being that is unchangeable; transness proposes that one is capable of realising and embodying change that runs deep.

Another problem – that emerges when support or solidarity seems performative – is alienation – which can push people who are actually the targets of hegemony and fascists out of organising and communities. It takes a particular form of strength and resilience to say, 'hey, this solidarity is in fact *not that helpful* – we need to have more nuanced exchanges in which we can develop understandings and practices over time'. For instance, the statement 'trans women are women', might be well intended, proposing 'women' as a trans-inclusive category, but can have the effect of assimilating and reducing feminist and trans critiques of the category of woman itself.[22] Sometimes, public statements are aimed at an abstract or imaginary public (for instance, at a protest), rather than at the individuals you are building your world with. Direct speech, written messages, and practices that are demonstrative are all better for communicating with those you are world-travelling with; and in a dehumanising world where much of our communication may occur through social media owned by huge corporations (even if these platforms have at times become virtual spaces for revolutionary and radical organising), we don't assume that knowing this is a given. To sustain collective learning is hard when people are tired and broken from the general state of oppression and violence, and from having to be resilient all the fucking time. Being hurt is personal, while enacting violence often results from indifference or distance.

This work of solidarity emerges from radical transfeminist and anti-colonial action groups, like STAR, who laid bare the connections between colonial violence, prisons, their lived conditions, and pathways to liberation.[23] A relational theory of trans thinks trans through affinity with social forms.[24] At its best, trans activity forms an ethics that aims to escape the toxic relationalities of patriarchy and deathly hierarchies of capitalism. It dispels hostile environments to shared spaces with a fuller sense of openness that allows exploration and a host of different sensations.

That we can make our worlds together doesn't require us to be the same; ethics is, after all, a negotiation of difference. Such a negotiation shapes an intimacy that does not rely on the formalised structures that organise hegemonic life, and put people in boxes, so to speak. Healing separation requires a shift in the physics of group-making. This means that the fundamental constituents, such as identity, that order structures of (anti-)sociality need to shift because these arrangements maintain existing forms.[25] Such shifts happen in part by opening up spaces for connection, which can happen by collective organising, or sharing workspaces, universities, community centres, and clubs. Collective forms do not come into existence because of a maximum of knowledge exchange, but because the focus is less on knowing 'what' and more on knowing 'how' (to be around each other and do things differently), and knowing 'when' to do something.[26] The crucial point of this shift is that the *how* of doing things together and making sure people stay connected can inform the *when* of ensuring that social forms do not address marginalisation 'last', in favour of a 'general' approach.[27] To have been people's first trans lover, partner, friend, collaborator, or colleague is part of changing community attitudes towards an openness to trans people – even if this can come with strenuous moments for trans people involved.[28] These intimacies, so to say, can be more or less literal, yet they do inform responses to our environment and shift discussions from academic (in a broad sense of the word) to more ethically informed practices, and that also means having learnt just to be around someone: to de-marginalise. Every struggle takes place at the heart,[29] and it takes time for collectives to incorporate these lessons with generosity on all sides: patience with learners, openness to support perspectives one might not understand, and navigating slip-ups, in the end solidarity is about undoing separability and disbanding hierarchies.

Practices are often messy, and there is no harmonious utopia awaiting at the end. A trans ethics acknowledges the messiness, the friction, the rise and fall of forms, and the social understanding that comes with them. It doesn't do this because of an innate characteristic 'because we are trans'; but because trans plurality taught us that engagement with ethics needs to be dynamic: people are not stuck in one spot, and the trans umbrella is broad. When difficult moments in movements are smothered in perfection and critique, movements peter out and agents find themselves isolated in unworkable individualisations of action. Yet, when building movements as collective practices that make new ways to flow, we can see that collectivising is not bound to a single form of organising: practices are messy. As we discussed in Chapter 2 femme work in organising consists often in working through relations and frictions. Friction is key to finding form and direction. Movements can form new ways to be with the world, but only through the absence of management[30] can collective transformation occur.

The focus on practice shows us how new social movements emerge from friction. María Lugones again offers key insights to address this situation by indicating the differences between forms of friction. Lugones draws a two-stage line through whiteness, as the colonial relation, and then through patriarchy. Lugones puts the question first to disband (institutionalised) hierarchy (the colonial disposition) and then to disband purification (the patriarchal relation).[31] While these refusals are not necessarily sequential, they offer an insight into relationality. The colonial disposition inhibits relationality and replaces it with hierarchy, while the patriarchal drive to maximise its own logic, understood as purification of collectives, rests on a sense of controlled attachment. In the inverse, these insights offer a frame for the space of solidarity. Instead of institutions, we can switch hierarchised indifference for the possibility of contextual relationality. Patriarchy, with its single logic that orders relationality, can be shifted towards pluralist approaches to making worlds. Solidarity can be understood as the space in which worlds meet and engage without hierarchy or purification. This also means, by way of Arturo Escobar, that it is not the space where sleeves are rolled up and problems solved.[32] Despite the perhaps attractive workerist imaginary, solidarity consists of being present without taking it upon yourself to make problems go away, and in that move impose a single world on differing lived realities.

LISTENING, LIVING, AND STRATEGISING TO DISSOLVE SEPARABILITY

Practice-based ethics contributes to collectivity with a mindset that holds difference as complementary. Ruth Wilson Gilmore might call this mindset *syncretism* or Gloria Anzaldúa might term it *hybrid*.[33] A syncretic practice uses comparison to create connections and stretch questions from the local to conceptual levels. This makes a practice-based ethics environmental and collective, resisting deferral to hierarchical structures of expertise, while holding space for external knowledge. This material approach addresses environments as atmospheres that people contribute to, whether they are intentional or not – in contrast to the hostile atmospheres created by media, normative assumptions, and institutional duress. It invites resistance to such normative encroachment.

In this practice-based ethics, identity is not static and a marker of a hierarchical structure, but historical/hirstorical. In a forward-looking temporality, a set of principles determines and stabilises future possibilities, shaping *what* one will be in the future, and making identity a projection of current social hierarchies. Racial and gendered hierarchies are good examples: as fundamental organising principles of a system of accumulation, they project into the future in which groups are relegated to the realms of extraction. This stabilisation of identity, furthermore, delimits what institutional transformation can look like, because, as we discussed before, institutions protect both hierarchy and accumulation. In contrast, a historical reading (a backwards-looking temporality) suggests identities hold knowledge that has been built up under consecutive systems of duress and resistance. Identities store insights, knowledge, and practices that inform current ethics and insurgencies against duress. (In a commodified approach to identity, reducing identity to a category and a set of signifiers, these insights, knowledges, histories and practices are rendered out of view.)[34] A syncretic approach relies on these memories and histories to bring different strategies and insights together, to overcome the hostilities that narrow descriptions and stabilisations of difference impose on organising.[35]

While planning our way out of the margins,[36] we sense different socialities, including what reverberates in languages not our own. Sensory openness is key to knowing what we can hold, and how we can be held, when we do not rely on a single form of life to situate us. Bodily being is not 'uncritical', as idealist approaches will have it, but there is a risk when working from our embedded selves of reinforcing a single pattern of life and purifying it.[37] Síle Darragh, former Political Prisoner interned at Armagh Goal, reflects that 'You need to bring people with you and you don't just need to bring your own people with you: you need to be able to reach out'.[38] Indeed, Ruthie Gilmore warns not to use 'comparison to create distances rather than alliances'.[39] We do not solely rely on what we know, but draw on curiosity. Perry Zurn and Arjuna Shankar write 'at its best, curiosity fuels an openness to difference and a drive towards innovation that together equip us to pursue a more intellectually vibrant and equitable world'.[40] These combined insights help us to remain curious about practices that shed light on who we are becoming *with* and how our own becoming takes place. In this sense, solidarity entails the willingness to give up the exclusivity of one's own perspective and be informed by points of view that might seem removed. Here, solidarity means that we are asked to rethink which foundations are embedded in our perspective. Secular writers sometimes contrast their perspective 'without a coherent worldview' to religious members of society, who apparently get coherence from their religion.[41] Often, this view hides commitments that are taken for granted, such as a certain functioning of bureaucracy and hierarchy. Rather than assume perspectives, AnaLouisa Keating offers '[t]heir willingness to actively engage in open conversations about differences enables them to insist on commonalities without assuming that their experiences, histories, ideas, or traits are identical with those of others'.[42] Keating discusses an openness to expose stereotypes, labels, and imaginary sameness, and 20 years down the line, we are working in this lineage of difference without separability. Solidarity which emerges from contrasting perspectives is often self-taught in the sense that it does not follow a script but allows connections to unfurl and connections emerge out of fragments. It can feel slightly chaotic because it doesn't follow disciplinary patterns. Practical solidarity can draw inspiration from anywhere because the important factor is relevance, rather than disciplinary boundaries.[43] A solidarity based on openness is slow-grown and constantly shifting. Openness requires a constant return to embodied living, steering away from ideological approaches.

Practices that work to dissolve the social, material, and legal divisions encoded between us[44] are not necessarily easy or straightforward. They also involve reflecting upon, remaking and unmaking our social lives within which wealth, skills, labour, and other resources get pooled and may end up oriented towards reproducing hegemony. Our everyday interactions sit within and upon the structures and mechanics of separability – indeed, we are all involved in reproducing particular social exclusions, be they based on languages or citizenship or dominant ethnicities or other norms. We can involve ourselves in their refusal and unmaking, and in fabricating alternatives – ceasing to labour in the service of white supremacy, or capital, or institutional transphobia, and reorienting our labour and skills towards spaces of possibility – although this won't happen without eking out time and capacity for transformative practices.

When communities and organisations are structured around (categorical) identities and shared traits in otherwise homogenous contexts (think cities that are seemingly not so diverse), other norms remain present and unspoken within the cultures of such groups. In Europe, one such problem is whiteness; in queer spaces, even diverse ones, cisnormativity may be another. These norms may be present and unspoken, unaddressed and without consideration until someone from outside of the fray raises their voice. Responses to such social marginalisation even with radical communities or minoritised communities – and often for the right reasons – has been to take up autonomous organising, leaving white people to make their own mistakes in unreflective organisations (because, as Black and Brown people, we had been burnt by trying to work in them); for the women to split from the men, for they refuse to check their misogyny; for the queers to not work with the straights, as they don't get the particular ways our lives cohere through our desires; and for the transfeminine folks to give up on unaddressed transmisogyny within other minority communities, including trans and non-binary communities. That people break away along social fault lines of racialisation, misogyny, trans, and queerness, is telling of pressures faced. However, homogeneity does not provide safety. Conflicts, pressures, and frictions in such break-away collectives are equally present. A lack of generosity from empowered individuals who foreclose social relations through the imposition of reductive dynamics may create the necessity to withdraw from a collective gathering.[45] Separability is at its most reductive when it starts to be posited as a basis for arranging social dynamics: splitting people into perceived categories that follow social fault lines. At that moment, there might be a clear class dynamic at play: ordering the world through exclusion in accordance with assumed sameness. This is markedly clear by the absence of certain categories: for instance, rurality or class, including self-sorting categories.

It takes active intervention, careful construction, curation and planning, and doing interpersonal groundwork, to undo traces of dominant norms in our social worlds, even from within marginalised communities.[46] Acting outside of one's comfort zone, not just for diversity or inclusion as per the neoliberal multiculturalist model, but from an ethics that shares skills and resources and that is open to constructive study, requires learning from different movements – forging and deepening connections across difference. One powerful example has been in public conferences organised by SWARM (Sex Worker Activism and Rights Movement) in the UK in the late 2010s, which set out to construct intersectional panels, which led to deepening understandings of shared struggles across differences with regard to international decriminalisation of sex work, abortion activism, and healthcare access and legal status more broadly.[47] Starting from elaborate multiplicities broadens the scope of the conversations, and the shared work to be done to forge collaborative imaginaries. *Structures* will not change through individual actions – but individual actions can chip away at the divisions that cohere around our social lives, collectives and organisations, to build better understandings of power, exclusion and violence through our everyday practices in order to loosen the everyday stranglehold of racial capitalism.

Worlds that intermix, brushing up against each other, over social divides, allow for the sharing of knowledge, resources, and possibilities. It doesn't have to involve befriending everyone, but it does mean reducing the climate of hostility and aggression enculturated in our interactions. In the intermeshing of collectives, we can build relations and grounded practices to counter tenets of separation; alternate tools may be forged to relieve the pressures of hegemonic structures and oppressions or dismantle them in a different manner. But all of this requires agency and (collective) intentionality – challenging how we are 'supposed' to behave in a society obedient to capital and the nation-state. Through reaching out of the mire of the sociality of the nation-state, we may build better understandings of problems – some shared, others not – and work to externalise them out of the separations imposed by nation-states.

In underlining the importance of remaining open, we emphasise an aptitude that has a particular resonance regarding transness and gender non-conformity. It is through holding open dialogues, spaces of learning, and perspectives to what has been othered, or marked 'deviant' or 'alien', that one may encounter how these otherwise knowledges or practices connect within oneself. For instance, most trans people who have been out as trans will be able to recall interpersonal connections and friendships that walk the fine lines of curiosity regarding gender non-conformity – trying to not stray into the fetishistic, while remaining interested, if understated and *not explicit*. In these friendships or connections, we find that over time, the fixity of gender for the person who is curious may be released – as they open themselves towards stepping away from the hegemony of norms that may have surrounded them, or the gender roles that have been imposed upon them.

SOLIDARITY (FOR THE LOVE OF FRICTION) AND AGENCY

As part of our transfeminism, we work on not being constrained by our *techne* (our enculturated and reworked modes of making connection), our languages, and our lived forms. We flow with the thought that 'social life is not a relation between things, but is rather, the field of rub and rupture that works, while being the work of, no one, nothing, in its absolute richness'.[48] With a sense of openness, we hold and embrace friction and rub as the meeting point, the meaning of relation moves from immobilisation in social positions towards the improvisational interplay with the field of being – the garden of life that we are growing in. We are constituted by our meetings, as much as we are trying to direct our becoming. Stephanie Camp notes that before the rise of a strong state, everyday conflicts over everyday practices were especially important.[49] In contemporary times, with states and corporations providing top-down orderings, confrontations have taken on another register. Rather than a direct clash between different people living in an area, protests have become actions that aim to influence policies, and consequently are indirect in nature. In the corporate and bureaucratic orderings of the con-temporary state, 'influence groups' push policymakers, and policy shapes space. This is the form of change pursued by the Non-Profit or NGO Industrial Complex.[50] However, in spaces of solidarity, con-frontation works more like the old model, where friction is a direct negotiation. Conflicts are not a sign of breakdown, but rather a sign of negotiations about space taking place. Rebecca Subar phrases it as follows: 'conflict is when your people want something, and the other side isn't giving it up'.[51] Stuart Hall adds that crisis is when a current form of life cannot be reproduced.[52] In direct conflicts with each other, the aim is perhaps not to win, but to reshape space together. The points of friction are the points where, for instance, insights about the direction of movements clash, perceptions mismatch, but also when hierarchies are brought in that disrupt connection. Some of these clashes need to be lived, rather than won, because these clashes can create connection, rather than separation. Some clashes are about disrupting social hierarchies, but not every clash is reducible to hierarchy.

One such division at present is a supposed cis/trans binary, which in the anglophone political context has been working to separate trans and non-binary people into a 'third gender' (of sorts), and/or attempting to legislate trans people out of public life and record (as discussed in Chapter 3). A social effect is that this tries to prevent people from 'crossing the divide' through identification *with* us. In practice, our actual lives, our worlds, do not contain such straightforward divisions – most trans people likely conduct their everyday lives living and working with non-trans people. Many non-trans people will know someone who is trans, but on what terms that person is *in their lives* can't really be specified generally. And if the media and state operate through the reiteration of narratives and bureaucracy that endeavour to objectify or dehumanise trans and non-binary people, everyday exclusion is essential for this to work – for there to be no transfeminist dialogic presence; to foreclose the possibility of conversations that address common problems, experiences, and practices among trans and non-trans people, between transfeminists and feminists more broadly. In practice, we may all be trying to work towards dismantling carceral and other apparatuses of duress in our lives, combatting misogynistic violence (without involving the police), ensuring that we can access the healthcare we need to survive (or live better), surviving accessing healthcare or living with the outcomes of these effects. These conflicts can accelerate reflection – and in the renewed intimacy of meeting, people need to be confronted with assumptions, and afterwards there should be a notable shift in behaviour and use of agency.[53]

Why do we emphasise agency when we think about solidarity? Is solidarity not reaching out to people in situations, which *you* might not be able to do something about; and in times of crisis, allowing people to reach in? Robin Kelley, in a brilliant talk given at LSE in London, made the argument that solidarity is working for *total* liberation.[54] This means in part that one works based on where one finds oneself, in connection to the surroundings one is in. Solidarity entails enabling one's actions and those of others, creating a context to build power, presence, and possibility. It means also that one questions what tools (or methods, or forms) one uses to approach organising and who these tools benefit: for who do they keep worlds open, and for who do they close them? Complicity asks questions about entanglement and brings to one's attention resistance and action against forms of organisation. Sometimes this means protesting content, or the absence of it, and sometimes it means disrupting forms of organisation, which can take many direct and indirect forms in itself. Reminding ourselves of Zurn and Shankar who present curiosity as counterpoint to indifference and imposition, we find forms of solidarity that rest on difference without separability. In the face of objectification and marginalisation within the dynamics and affective economies of separability, solidarity creates vibrations that allow one to break out of patterns of thought and feeling which may otherwise keep one stuck in commitments that benefit the status quo. Breaking indifference by means of openness allows one to be touched by situations of immiseration, injustice, and hierarchy. It entails cultivating and being animated by a sense of empathy in the unbearable light of injustice; it may entail an active practice, in Hartman's words, of loving what is not loved.[55] Through these senses of feeling, (which are hopefully grounding, and need to not be exiled toward hopelessness), to establish or undertake concrete action. Not all actions that comprise solidarity are directly relational, but they are informed by a sense of connection. For instance, some forms of redistribution of material resources are not immediate; and the unlearning of assumptions requires self-study. However, solidarity as activity towards total liberation needs collective action and thus needs greater relationalities. We hold that these should be non-hierarchical to allow space for different focus points and different strategies, and not subsuming different struggles under a single form of action.

A focus on agency and solidarity takes the pressure off a focus on knowledge (i.e. subjectivity), which in turn enables holding various perspectives at the same time. Shifting the primacy in social change from knowledge to action alleviates the need to have a single, coherent vision of what liberation and oppression look like. This might lead to a collective of 'intimacies', using Jen Nash's term[56] – where different approaches that address separability can come together as active solidarity. Such active solidarities can take the form of delightfully autodidactic approaches that freely draw from different sources, and are not subject to disciplinary constraints, an improvisation that keeps patriarchy on the backfoot. A solidarity freed from disciplinary registers can cooperate across imposed boundaries, and it remains solidarity as long as it aims at total liberation.

VANQUISHING VIOLENCE WITH ABOLITIONIST PRACTICES

As we argued in Chapter 4, we are shaping lived realities, rather than just living in subjugation according to another's image of us, yet the projections we live through remain steady. The bitter experiences our lives include having been subject to violence, rape, sexual harassment, and a transgression of human rights (whatever you think about rights, this is still indicative of a significant violence) – *and yet* in the mainstream press (not just the conservative papers) trans people are still depicted as a threat and perpetrators of violence. Still, resentment will keep us estranged from collectivity. Anti-trans discourses work to reaffirm and reproduce affective economies of separability – the dehumanisation, villainisation, objectification, and othering of trans women, and trans and non-binary people more broadly, in order to exile or outlaw us from society. We don't find it surprising that anti-trans discourses focus on prisons and toilets: enclosed spaces that isolate us from the ways we live. The imagery of isolation in the ways anti-trans activists write about us shows what they want with us: to isolate people from each other, which makes us controllable, and to keep us outside of spaces where encounters are possible, interrupting as much connection as possible. This is why anti-trans activists do not mind trans toilets: as long as we are kept apart, we can be locked out. Our doing time, inside and outside prisons (currently there are six trans women in women's prisons in the UK)[57] means that many of us are isolated in our rooms, houses, and homes, because of this violent atmosphere and interrupted socialities.

We have discussed how the practice of transformation is not without risk. Violence and duress are the dominant modes of 'putting people back in their place'. Sometimes this means people are bullied out of public spheres. In resistance movements we find rape culture, which is a way of signalling that the feminist revolution is not welcome here. And yet, knowing those risks and sticking together while practising community safety by broadening our connections to each other is the way to make a future. Because of the violence and duress that we have seen, experienced, and heard, we propose a transfeminist ethics that refuses institutionalised powers that create punishment. Instead, we risk ourselves by being vulnerable and keeping each other safe. The risks of vulnerability come in another register, as some of us might not be used to sharing our fears and worries, and are afraid of judgement. The intimate connection between risk, vulnerability, and transformation is sometimes used against collectives, but allows for our collective strengths to come out.

Trans femme lives face the institutionalised demotion of transness, accompanied by femmephobia, misogyny, and further intersecting forms of duress. This means that there is no 'it gets better (and more toxic too)' that is bestowed by hegemonic structures. However, women can also be agents of violence, which is often overlooked in feminist theory. Such violence has received some attention in recent years, for instance, through the figure of the 'Karen' – the white woman who calls the police.[58] The experience in trans lives of women attacking trans existence calls into question automatic solidarity through gender. The harassment of (bourgeois, poor, Black, Brown, white, queer, lesbian) women by (bourgeois, poor, Black, Brown, white, queer, lesbian) women has forever taken the form of doubting someone's womanhood – and thus transmisogyny is misogyny.[59] It is not the enforcement of the gender binary that creates connection. When people are willing to pause their intuitions and be open to listening, sharing, and affirming events, perspectives, and actions in people's lives, what is found are overlaps, the excitement of understanding the world in a new manner, and a willingness to create new forms of living together. Feminism remains necessary, but it needs to overcome its harassment of sex workers, trans people, queers, the poor, single mothers, immigrants, people of colour, working classes, and so on, with claims that marginalised people undermine the position of the complainant.[60] Some people refuse to take on the term feminist as a result (one of us used to be one of them). And yet, the term helpfully reminds us of lineages that have attempted to make new intimate relations from which new worlds can emerge.

We do not think that trans people are immune from being implicated in violence. They can be for different reasons – sometimes due to trauma and incorporated violence, and sometimes because learning and healing still needs to happen. However, debates become lopsided, as prejudices, like every prejudice, are targeted to perpetuate hegemonic forms of harm. Ana-Maurine Lara writes that 'healing from our own personal experiences is not just a matter of personal health, healing is also a matter of social change.'[61] Healing from personal experiences of being harmed is hindered by ongoing perpetuations of violence to us and around us. As evident as that rephrase may sound, it is also informative for questions about how we want to live *now*, and what this asks from us while residing in a world where our membership is in question. It asks us to question, in Lara's words, 'how prepared we are to deal with the fallout from our personal experience with violence.'[62] Resentment is harming myself and the communities I am in, and it will also hinder seeing how I perpetuate violence and have perpetrated harm in the past. Still, the feeling of resentment isn't just in imaginations. Misrecognition is harm, it is a form of erasure, and it is invisibilising and in that sense painful. *However*, trying to stage a change in public debate based on resentment leads to a victim-led plea that will hinder the work of community-making and personal healing. Resentment makes people judgemental and closed off, which is how hierarchy and hegemony wants us to be. It takes effort to rise above the alarmist announcements in media and public spaces, and to keep reaching out to people who are open to reworking public understanding and to vanquishing (in Rebecca Subar's words) a certain form of patriarchal and transphobic debate. My healing of resentment is for myself, for the people around me, and hopefully something that in my communities is dealt with, with care. In the future we want to live already, it requires dealing with these sentiments to build something in which we can thrive. At the same time, facing this resentment is part of facing our own contributions to harm and the actions it makes us do, both societal, personal, and interpersonal, which is an ongoing reality in our communities. It requires facing the energy drain that is imposed on us, in trying to deal with this, but also facing when we are lashing out at people close to us.

Abolition guides us through dealing with resentment, to understanding our needs to have a place, as well as a voice in our communities, worlds and collectives. Demanding subjection to our views is not a way to get to transformative justice. The everyday intentions, relations and commitments that abolitionist feminists adopt are not designed to be taken up in a monolithic fashion – they are actions infused with the belief that we can live in manners that negate and reduce the impact of injustice. If we focus on outcomes and effects of structural dynamics of violence, and the unwillingness to give up power, we may work to intervene in the sources of harm, to intervene in the relations that cause harm, while orienting collectively towards reparative new practices. To open up helps to stage the developing ground for abolitionist ethics. We build together and fight outside. Justice is reached by the means of coming together, but not by the defeat of our 'enemies'. The win (in case you are looking for such a term) is that people become more

open and active in abolitionist practices. Alisa Bierria offers 'Abolitionist strategy that aspires to *teach* requires rigour in two things: its
truth and its capacity to produce an opening for others to meaningfully connect with that truth.'[63] When those that we need to fight are
to become active in abolition, it invites people to change their ways.
The less time we have to spend in the way we want, the more the
anti-trans movement gains. The far-right – and people with institutional power – have to deny our truths because, to them, they
are unbearable. Practices, however, are less easily denied (requiring surveillance and criminalisation). New practices become forms
of justice.

Concretely, one of the ways to orient our collective endeavours
around anti-violence is centring community safety. In recent years
(especially since 2017), anti-transphobic and anti-fascist feminist
organising has coalesced around challenging TERF platforms and
spaces. While these interventions are important, practices change
when prioritising the safety needs of marginalised trans people,
including trans sex workers, migrants, Black and Brown folks, trans
femmes and women, gender non-conforming people, and queers
and women more broadly. Prioritising safety needs is a direct and
action-oriented challenge to our dehumanisation and counters the
dismissal of our exclusion from social life and its attendant affective economies. It challenges climates that enable transfemicide[64]
and the conditions in which direct and indirect transmisogynist and
transphobic harm manifest. It also challenges the use of policing in
a manner that can support people who have experienced incarceration and people on the inside. Community safety, and collective
defence as a form of self-defence, are practices which may range
from physical training, providing safety supplies, moving through
the world or travelling together, etc. It is work that builds and maintains a qualitative and direct understanding of issues, problems or
situations that may arise in the particularities of the work we do and
the lives we lead, or may wish to lead.

Truth and trust are necessary in a struggle, as Ana-Maurine Lara
highlights in a discussion dedicated specifically to partner abuse in

queer (of colour) communities, truthfulness and trust as helping us grow stronger. Here it needs to be noted that such truthfulness and trust have limited use in fighting against oppression, but it *needs* to be worked on in communities that carry the fight. Lara offers that 'truthfulness with each other can lay the foundations for revolutionary consciousness, and for resolving the effects of abuse'.[65] Truthfulness is the driver for *learning* how to do this, where the term learning is of key importance – both in our work to deal with ourselves and the effects of violence; the violence of which we have been perpetrators as well as having been the harmed person. This means that hopes for a hasty resolution where there's a discursive driver of change (the way we talk about what should have been) is not necessarily the best emphasis, because the embodied driver for change requires a different pace: one with more generosity, kindness, and also truthful accountability.

THE LONG HAUL

To underscore how the longer term could take form, we focus on patterns in activist activity; from learning in movement work, action-orientation, and building solidarity, to ways of knowing ourselves as participants in collective movements.

Solidarity shapes forms of justice that support communities. Community spaces are needed to come together after stressful moments, which is a part of movement work. In these spaces hyper-vigilance and interpersonal and intimate violence are testimony to the stress of received violence. The circle is not yet broken, but solidarity work is dealing with it and shaping a space for connection. The loss of many community spaces that are collectively organised, for instance, squats and social centres, has been a huge setback for movement work. There's no need to wax lyrical with nostalgia over what has been lost to see that the squat movement provided a foundation for many initiatives that supported solidarity work. The movement functioned also as a low-key ethical maintenance of those foundations, even if part of the work of movements is to re-learn over and over the same lessons in different generations. Yet,

Lara notes that foundations built by our generation were not maintained.[66] However, we also see that lessons need to be re-learnt at various moments as part of a pattern of refusing hegemonic tools for dealing with situations. Relearning allows people to embody alternative forms. We need to practice insights that emerge from movements, sometimes with the support of mentorship, but it is also important to face oneself in difficult situations and figure out how things work. Shira Hassan's proposal to practice Liberatory Harm Reduction – to curb negative impacts while not succumbing to either harm or control, is a way to view conflicts in communities too.[67] We need to work to curb damage, create space for relationality and liberation, but we cannot hope to create a community in which conflicts never do harm without collapsing into a rule-driven and policed environment (which comes with its own harms).[68] It is better to face the harm and curb its impact, than pretend we can manage to avoid it altogether. This means we need to build skills in dealing with conflict, harm, and its consequences.

Another part of building movements is to organise around issues that allow for channelling of collective energy, and formulating creative responses in practice. The response to a particular event can galvanise and activate a movement, in either transformative or reactionary directions. Responses to events do not necessarily turn into long-term social transformation, and whether this work energises or drains the actors within is not a given. Right-wing movements and media outlets have created a huge capacity for anger-focus, yet their game is not to 'solve' problems, but to keep the anger going, from one to the other topic. The perpetual cycle of anger and aggravation shapes an audience that is escalating its demands for more aggressive solutions. A left-wing strategy of openness and collective reflection does not always match this tone, because solidarity runs in another track: a track of connection, camaraderie, grief, joy (hopefully), and engaged personal, social change, rather than angry dismissal. Solidarity has a longer breath, but is also more vulnerable.

Bodies, when given space to breathe, often calm down. This is useful to know, for instance, when you're in a conflict and want to change the situation: give some room and let some of the tension evaporate.[69] Another situation in which this can be observed is in an actual fight, when a body feels less threatened, it lets go of some tension and the fight slows. It takes training to keep speeding up the body and continue pushing your opponent. We can see similar patterns in movement organising: it takes a longer-term focus to keep people engaged. Especially when people feel they've won something, calm often ensues. Rebecca Subar reflects on this in the wake of the 2008 Obama election: rather than going into the streets, many organisers calmed down and reviewed the policies of the new administration.[70] Similarly, experience with union organising shows that local victories can slacken the energy of members of a branch. While we can understand this as justified and a shift from fighting energy to negotiating energy, we can also see how such a lessening of energy requires different strategies to keep people engaged, and switching from (short-term) goal to goal is not always the best way forward.

And yet, collectives that coalesce around an activity (such a collective art-making) often have room for reflection on oneself or group processes. Collectives that are meant to share experiences (such as consciousness-raising groups) are not necessarily strong in moving to action-orientation, but display a tendency to homogenise, because the shared consciousness creates the group.[71] A task orientation, for instance, growing carrots, or shopping for people who are house bound, can help bring people together, without a focus on how your experiences determine you. Actions allow for mixed collectives. With the activity providing the bond, experience-sharing can flow in an open form. Collectives that move between actions and consciousness-raising need to address this flow between the different orientations to keep people engaged. Sometimes, this can happen by moving activity out of one's direct interests, such as working in solidarity.

In our contemporary debates, it is easy to observe affinity rushing along a vertical axis: about learning from 'the most oppressed', partly through the language of intersectionality.[72] To put a hand in my own pocket: from (para-)academics to the wretched of the earth, so to say. This doesn't mean that the 'wretched' feel the same sense of affinity with the social pressures I receive in my position, and I should be very aware of that.[73] Accountability for struggles that are not academic in nature can forge bonds between communities and isolated academics, which undoes the (self-)importance of academic work at the same time as embedding thinkers outside the demands of the institution.[74] Practices of solidarity create mutuality – the moment I start to work *in* communities, mutuality grows around the activities we are engaged in, but this doesn't mean our lives are the same.

Our ethics manifests in thinking about how we live processes from the inside.[75] As Mariame Kaba explains, we are used to looking at processes of oppression from the outside, but these systems live within us, and we are not used to looking at them from the inside. Accountability to collectives outside the academy counters the 'zero point epistemology' that is located in the mind only, and which the Western academy relies on.[76] Academic epistemologies that lay claim to be the proper forms of knowledge, ground a manner of knowing in a manner that is not grounded at all: it is disembedded and disembodied and holds allegiance to a formal structure while it avoids reviewing whether some truths are perhaps local. That this way of knowing is the result of formal procedures in research and presentation is sufficient for its validity. In contrast, knowing can also emerge from the heart and body, with a sensory openness, that draws its insights from where one is active, often in addition to a scattering of sources that are deemed relevant for the point of struggle.[77] This knowing acknowledges its locality and is thus accountable as a matter of ingrained perspective. The accountability that transformative justice relies on links to this manner of knowing because it asks not how the structures operate, but how do we operate in our environments.[78] Our complicities in systems of oppression may be glossed over when we beeline to claim our space within a marginalised, categorical identity – uncritically flattening the nuance of its inflexion. While Kaba reflects that one cannot force people to be accountable to others, similarly one cannot force people to face their position as an internal process – positionality is quite often stated as a list of externalised categories, which ends the reflection.[79] Solidarity becomes possible by shifting from affinity to activity. And that shift can take place under a critical practice of love – to open up to who is not you, or like you, and widening your sensorium and curiosity to transform the manner in which our world is experienced. H.L.T. Quan notes: 'it is troubling that we rarely frame mass mobilisation as a desire for friendship, or foreground love as a motivation for movement formation.'[80]

TRANSFEMINIST PROPOSALS FOR LOVE

The present is a time of ubiquitous and powerful aphorisms and dialogues on self-love, which can help with self-affirmation in the face of harm and denigration. The trouble is that they are also fed to us by a neoliberal individualism that itself retrenches hierarchies, especially of wealth, literally leaving marginalised folks to fend for themselves. In Chapter 2, we discussed affective economies as a framework for understanding how our deep emotions and our openness tend to get pooled – in the relationships, chosen and assigned families, communities and sometimes the struggles our lives are situated within (maybe sometimes in our jobs too). If one was to describe a transfeminist love-politics – responding to the affective, social, economic, bureaucratic circuits that marginalise trans life – we could turn to the forms of trans, femme, and queer collectivity that explicitly entail pooling our love for each other. As Kai Cheng Thom vividly describes in *I Hope We Choose Love*, in the eye of the storm of the everyday violence of 'gendered and racialised laws and social norms [that] dictate almost every aspect of society [...] [w]e are forced to redefine happiness as loving ourselves on our own terms.'[81] Thom emphasises that this is '[t]he kind of happiness that is only found at the centre of a whirlwind, in the arms of your community'. This is a mutuality that can provide gender euphoria, can bear grief and, hopefully, support each other through the harms and violences wherever we may experience them. The collective forms of queer, trans, sex worker and street homeless, care or social reproduction that Nat has written about elsewhere, such as Sylvia Rivera and Marsha P. Johnson's STAR House, may be necessary for trans and queer survival and life in general,[82] but the social conditions that give rise to their necessity are also what we are trying to transform – work that trans and queer folks can by no means do alone. It is the dynamics of separability that enclose (around) our worlds, that leave us to tend to each other with (sometimes extreme) degrees of harm and trauma that have accumulated in us and in our communities, alongside limited resources.[83]

The proposition of transness as a movement away from an unchosen starting place towards something else comes with an opening up towards expression. If transness works through forms of love – a self-love, community love, love of the play of gender or the disruption of norms – it is a form of love where we can bring more of ourselves than the norms of gender would otherwise allow us; it is a love that calls for growth, for becoming. A love that encourages a 'recognition' of the potential trajectories we may take or desire with our ensouled bodyminds – acknowledging trans desire; a love that encourages us to believe in the propositions to come.

In her writing critically addressing Black feminist love-politics, Jennifer Nash emphasises the transformative possibilities in committing to mutual vulnerability and witnessing. 'Mutual vulnerability is marked by a commitment to unleashing the "sacred possibilities" between us, recognising our deep interdependency with each other, with the more-than-human world and the ecologies in which we live'.[84] Acting with love from this position understands that 'thriving requires our co-existence'; while vulnerability is, here drawing from Berlant and Butler, not simply about the potential of to be injured, but moreover undergirding the radical non-sovereignty of relations infused by love – 'vulnerability requires us to embrace that face that we can be – and often are – undone by each other'.[85] Such vulnerability, Nash writes, 'can take the form of grief and mourning, desire and ecstasy, solidarity and empathy, and mutual regard'.[86] Nash elsewhere considers June Jordan's writing on love as engendering of the Black public sphere, where the public sphere 'is a site where selves labouring to love – to orient their selves towards difference, towards transcending the self – join in a form of relationality'.[87] Nash underlines the insistence of Black feminist love-politics 'on transcending the self and producing new forms of political communities' – it is indicative of a willingness to change and be changed.[88] As the queers in the room, we remember that desire sits at the basis of the bonds and sociality that have animated much of Black feminist literature, cultural production and herstory.[89] Indeed, Audre Lorde argues, in her 1979 'The Master's Tools Will Never Dismantle the Master's House', that the desire for nurturance between women is 'redemptive', a locus of power, and that 'It is this real connection which is so feared by a patriarchal world'.[90]

Our proposal for embracing complicity, in and against affective economies and separability, encourages us to consider what degrees of openness to difference we actually live and practice. Does sexual racism, for instance,[91] propose that we are only open to those who fall into a framework of recognition grounded in, say, ethnic or cultural or gender sameness? If love is typically only forged between people who are alike, those who are like us – even given the animosity that we receive, as people marginalised by ability or race or gender, from others for our existence – what are we really open towards?[92] Love may enrich and animate us, when politics may leave us feeling drained; it can infuse the relationality that we need to dismantle the social divisions encouraged and engineered between us. With love, we may find reasons to stick beside each other, refuse disposability, and work through the harms towards remedy.[93] To echo Thom's words, a '[l]ove that cares about people more than ideas, that prizes each and every one of us as essential and indispensable'; a love that, in working towards reparative justice, 'asks the hard questions, that is ready to listen to the whole story and keep loving anyway'.[94]

Politicised approaches to love can manifest touch when it is prohibited or denied. In stories coming out of prison and from families of incarcerated members, 'the ruse of security' is used to block people from touching, and prisoners and outsiders are forced to talk through telecommunications – rather than meeting, holding hands, and hugging, where the space of touch is 'fundamentally about the right of incarcerated people to continue living, even in the shadows of so much death'.[95] Prisons, borders, and their manifestations in the outside world drive a wedge between our need and the ability to be touched, and in that touch, feel our vibrancy. Another thing that we learn from stories from prison is how abuse thrives on silence, and silence is maintained by the ability to look away, which is exploited by those in power – who endeavour to curb, limit, and restrict what is known or communicated. While stories carry sparks of knowledge across contexts, only if you let yourself be touched and move yourself into action does this knowledge land.[96]

Julietta Singh reminds us that Fanon described a form of revolutionary love as the bond that is forged on social and economic levels between two nonnormative bodies.[97] Sensitivity is a basis for that bond – not just openness: sensing the world beyond and between the map that narratives and language provides. Sensitivity is a 'bodily art' in Hawhee's term.[98] This is a situated gauging of indeterminacy in the moment, rather than having been taught what to do, and thus bypasses a rule-based mastery. This chimes with what María Lugones discusses as loving perception.[99] This kind of opening to the world and interlocuters in it, makes a demand on oneself in challenging 'critical' attitudes or demanding emotions. What Lugones offers is to open and listen without demanding specific forms of interaction that are already recognisable, 'cool', *du jour*, or sound in accordance with the 'right' way of saying things. An ensouled listening has space for connection beyond the confines of language-use, or affective codifications. AnaLouise Keating writes that this 'radical interrelatedness gives us – gives me – a responsibility to meet those I encounter with a sense of openness.'[100] In Keating's phrases this openness is not immediately towards a single person – or a domestic unit – but an openness towards all that lives. Perhaps we can open that further, by emphasising that we are open to all that vibrates.[101] We are influenced by our surroundings, even if they are not of our choosing, animated on levels beyond our direct perception, as we learnt from Eva Hayward in Chapter 1. What matters is that a respect for and openness towards vibrancy can be shared, even if it comes in different forms. It is about taking care and listening to people, animals, plants, and the earth in different modalities. As Gilmore states, 'abolition should be green. It has to take seriously environmental harm, environmental racism, and environmental degradation'.[102] Listening encourages making space to respond, and to understand what one is vibrating with, the anima that moves one, in and through the ensouled bodymind. Ethics is an openness to all we share the world with.

I'm sitting in a park with a friend. They muse, sighing, that sometimes they feel profoundly alienated from the way trans is discussed, which makes it hard to join a conversation about the potentiality that trans holds. Stepping away from an owned identity to explore what might be possible comes with a certain release (and occasionally relief). When identity is not seen as an internal and inalienable property, but as an external and a social force that needs to be navigated, it opens a space for identity to change and even to be more than one thing at the same time.[103] Drifting away from the grasp of power requires indeterminacy, but is greatly aided with a sense of responsibility for the world in which one finds oneself. To shape and contribute is not the same as autonomy, as we discussed in Chapter 4.[104] Instead, we wonder how to lovingly acknowledge the vibrancy around ourselves, and shape interconnectedly the world we are moving in together. We hold on to each other while we navigate and respond to what is happening – as outcomes are open, as management is not here to lock the park gates. Connection, which is neither universal nor general, shows the promise of a future, where conversations, like bodyminds, emerge and change.

TRANS JOY

In the end, it's all about the joy of living our lives and the pleasure of shaping them together. This joy celebrates our hirstories, presence, and future in the present – it actively reminds us of the possibility of turning relationships around and living something more truthful and honest, which enables a deeper connection to ourselves, each other, and our environment. The vibrant energy of our connections highlights the joy of making relations again into something new, fun, and nurturing, revealing the enclosures of normative gender as a cage that can be escaped. This is why trans is feminist – it remakes our lives into something we want to live, and this is why it is futurist

– we live in the world that needs to come into being in the present. Part of the pressure and rage directed at trans people is precisely because of the joy we can manifest. Our joy infuses the energy that we can direct at each other. Joy is both the shield that keeps hostility outside of our circle and the source of our openness.

The vulnerability in public spaces we inhabit is held by joy when our bodies are together. The community that gathered around the 2020 Black trans initiatives in New York of Qween Jean, Joela Rivera, and others came together for 'education, reinvigoration, for healing, for representation'.[105] It was a movement that worked to stage the contributions to Black liberation that had been ignored by social movements. The initiatives emerging from this focus on Black trans liberation inspired a 'vast diversity of the community' to come together.[106] Movement work is community love. Cindy Trinh, a photographer who recorded the 2020 get-togethers explains 'People that come [together] are bringing forth their bodies and their minds and coming from a place of wanting to learn and show that they care'.[107]

The connection between learning, gathering, and joy is intentional. Travis Alabanza writes 'Trans has always been about honesty and I will not let *them* rob me – *us* – of that'.[108] Travis reminds us that young trans people know things about gender way beyond their years, which is learning not only through experience, but because of this honesty; this openness to learn the world anew. Dominant theory will have us believe that such learning occurs through distancing and critical scrutiny, but our lives teach us that it comes just as much through doing, coming together, and loving the experiments we do together – never needing to know how things might end up. Yvonne Lebien suggests in a meditation about whether we should think the right thoughts 'I think we would be a lot happier if we stopped worrying so much about what we were thinking, because fundamentally thinking is not the most important part of the self. There is no important part: the self is a multitude of things happening in tandem'.[109] Our futures are forged through a multitude of our actions, thoughts, and practices leading us in our different ways – meeting each other in our multitudes with joy. Dreaming the directions we may take, and being open gives structure to the pleasure of learning, of connecting, and holding each other. *This learning connects our material lives with our dreams of futures that are not blocked by our internalised oppressions.* Dissolving the grip of these oppressions in the joy of seeing each other thrive, laugh, and love – seeing our connections across and beyond them.

While some trans joy might happen in public spaces, parties, or demonstrations, it is important not to overlook the pleasure of the everyday company of friends, lovers, and passers-by who join our living rooms and kitchen tables.[110] It's a pleasure of company, and there's also the pleasure of gendered connection, where people sometimes automatically connect in a way that feels right, even if it's just a chat about the price of food in the frozen aisle of the local supermarket. It is a moment that provides comfort against social pressures, duress and insecurities of showing up in public and not knowing what might happen. Travis writes about this as sometimes intermingled with guilt when the gendering is sexism, which also leads to solidarity from other women and femmes. Joy doesn't need to be pure – and there's more to life than defying expectations.[111] José Muñoz[112] introduces the term *disidentification* – a third term that is neither the imposition and assimilation by the norm, nor a direct form of resistance, but a way out that 'registers consequences' of identifications – to consider (aesthetic) practices filtered through humour or everyday subversion.[113] Disidentification indexes a form of play that filters pressures, recognisable forms, and associations, in defiance of the demand for compliance, including to be 'recognisable' and 'acceptable'. (It's also cathartic.) The joy that emerges from the play with the forms reveals the shallowness of our understandings that are trivialised under neoliberal strategies of 'inclusion'. And so, to play with forms, make them emerge in different manners, is to play the play of trans joy.

In the small acts of trans joy, we find an echo of the large acts of political liberation. Such feelings of connection and freedom might have been experienced at the Maidan, Gezi Park, Squat Culture, Anarchy in the UK in 1995, Occupy, and so on. Where the large movements faced collapse under violence, they took with them their seeds and a taste of freedom to live in another world. Quan writes '[these contemporary] movements do the work of living democracy, including destroying to build anew, all the while envisioning just futures'.[114] Trans joy is every day that tastes freedom in the wink, the smile, the joy of huddling in a corridor and sharing a moment, the pleasure of the parties, the kitchen tables or kitchen disco, and living rooms – which is not always a massive ground swell but is a barricade against normativity behind which we can connect.

MAKING TRANSFEMINIST FUTURES

Through joy, love, and solidarity, we build power, connection, and new and changed relations; our lives flourish. This is not an idealist project, or hope, or a future that might emerge after a struggle, but the everyday shift of sensibility, connections, and relations. Trans power is the power to change how we are in the world and what our worlds consist of. It is based on experience of making new relations to ourselves and each other, and what we build through these relations. Denaturalising social forms makes them visible, and shows them as fragile; it reveals social pressures and shows how much effort some put into maintaining forms that provide the safety of recognisability, or institutional stability, but perhaps are not worth the price. Binary genders, class, and racialisation are basic logics by which people navigate the world; even if it is not the world we want, it is the world we know. Trans life confronts normative stasis with the fact that it doesn't need to be so – that the world can shift, today. This trans-finding of forms experiments in gathering and letting go, which is echoed in the coming and going of terms one uses as self-descriptions. For some of our friends, allies, emerging and future trans people, and strangers, this freedom may feel exhilarating and like a relief – an aspect of gender euphoria. One is free to change forms – to a larger extent than if gendering (which are merely relations) has a definitive grip on social forms. As trans activists, writers and world-makers have been arguing since the 1990s, binary gendering doesn't have to be a tenet of social relations – releasing it throws gender, sexuality, social and thus a whole string of relational modes into relief.[115] This is perceived as a threat by transphobes and conservative feminists. A part of our work emerges from knowing that we don't need to reform the forms we live in; we can drop these forms and do something else, although such processes are slow and long-term. Refusal can happen today, growing something else takes time and takes each other. We already mentioned Anne-Marie Quinn's reminder that transformation needs slowness. Trans life adds that shifts are bodily and take time and that attentiveness needs to shift to those overlooked spaces, people, and connections. Genuine connection grows and might take years, yet our lives are what Saidiya Hartman would describe as practical proposals of *what-might-be*.[116] This also comes with the knowledge that we cannot change anybody else's form *for them*. But what we can do is extend an invitation to join us.

We invite all of you, as we have been invited by Gloria Anzaldúa, José Esteban Muñoz, María Lugones, Stefano Harney and Fred Moten, Jackie Wang, Ruth Pearce, Joy Mariama Smith, Marquis Bey, Travis Alabanza, Tourmaline, Kuchenga Shenjé, Raju Rage, Delilah Matrix, Chryssy Hunter, Jennifer Nash, Lola Olufemi, Nicole Sansone Ruiz, Jay Bernard, Vick Virtu, Sam Bourcier, Shuli Branson, Eric Stanley, Dean Spade, Arika, and many others. People should not struggle alone. Dissolving separability doesn't mean that transfeminism is only for trans people – as demonstrated by Hispanophone and Francophone transfeminisms[117] – but a mode of acting in the world that draws from the experience of living transformation.[118] Practices of sociality across difference are necessary for the transformations we will need to continue to live – our 'we' is not a 'we' of sameness, but the activities we share together. This engenders multiple practices and ways of coming together – many of them may start with eating together (we hope you'll come eat with us). Trying to live otherwise comes without a moral high ground, and it can only be done by figuring it out together.

Writing on the freedom literally dreamt by the family of Assata Shakur while she was imprisoned, Jackie Wang addresses how prophetic dreams come with 'the responsibility of the recipients [...] to make them real [...] acting so as to give them flesh.'[119] Bridging immediate social and material needs and our desires, collective dreaming – from the everyday to the essential to the utopian; the aesthetic, abstract and far-fetched to the ordinary and small – meets the concretisation of infrastructures, projects, spaces, and possibilities. Collective dreaming encourages experimentation, but its concretisation crucially requires us to lean into making material commitments – including ones with our bodies (again, a trans practice)[120] and financial ones. Towards worlds to live, eat and love in, to bear witness to each other in our lives; to tend our relationality and interdependency with each other and the world; to forge the promise of freedom that comes with jailbreak. In the mix, these practices manifest gratitude, actual recognition and substance, energising and lifting each other up, contra exploitation, denigrations and the logics of fetishism. Practices to unpick the foundations of the social order.

There are multiplicities of collective practices to create anarchic ensembles – from those led by shy radicals to those that voluminously reclaim public space, of different textures of rambunctiousness.[121] Particular collective practices may not fit everyone, or in the same way. Some are more playful, others more serious, some focus on small things, others on large overtly political projects. What practices of liberation share in common is that they are *out of the control* of authorities, whether gendered or the macro forces of institutionalised capture. We move together into transfeminist futurity to abolish structures of domination, incarceration, and separation. A driving refusal of compliance and deference opens a field for change, which enables people to bring their own potentialities and actualise them. We carry and grow our skills and knowledge in our multiplicities – some have experience connecting (with) strangers (inside and outside the prison system), some know how to organise groups, some know how to hold and make space, some know where the food comes from. We offer you the following questions, to take away and work through with your friends, collectives, with your siblings and yourselves: rather than inclusion for fear of being left out, how do transfeminist social spaces, exchanges, groups, organisations and collectives make our practices fuller, more 'real', and expansive, more possible? What forms of life and propositions for living can we enact together, as alternatives to the forms of precarity, overwork, overstimulation, and surveillance that neoliberal racial capitalism ensnares us within? What sustains our worlds and what do we need to keep them nourished? Futures emerge from getting together and learning to rely on each other – what will come will be formed and grown together. The logics of collective transformation breathes air into worlds for all of us.

Notes

INTRODUCTION

1. Stryker, *Transgender History*, 1; Bey, *Black Trans Feminism*.
2. Quan, *Become Ungovernable*, 166.
3. Common examples of flatting difference in the expression of sameness that we've witnessed in recent years include the rise and dominance of middle-class, educated whiteness in urban queer scenes, which we understand from Jin Haritaworn as itself a form of gentrification, which assume that educational access and Eurocentric ideas of gender are common for all participants. See Haritaworn, *Queer Lovers and Hateful Others*.
4. Arturo Escobar, María Lugones, and Denise Ferreira da Silva come to mind as anti-colonial thinkers; and Karl Marx, Theodor Adorno, Max Horkheimer, and Michel Serres as thinkers remaining in the European tradition.
5. Quijano, 'Coloniality of Power'.
6. This contrasts John Locke who claimed that prisoners were free because their minds were free. That is obviously untrue, even if we might agree that not every mind aligns with the pressures of the environment. A mind is simply not free when in prison: it is a mind in a prison after all and thus receives violence, duress, aggression and is held hostage by a state or private company. See van der Drift, 'Management and Rights' for discussion.
7. Kohn, *How Forests Think*.

CHAPTER 1: 'THEY WOULD PLANT
THE ROSE GARDEN THEMSELVES'

1. The authors thank Zia Álmos Joshua X for their take on Virginia Woolf's *Mrs Dalloway* (and Michael Cunningham's adaptation, *The Hours*), 'Ze would buy the flowers theirself'. An earlier version of parts of Chapter 1 and Chapter 3 have appeared as *Social Text* (Drift and Raha, 'They would plant the rose garden').

2. For discussions on feminisation of labour by gender non-conforming queers, see Hennessy, *Fires on the Border*; Raha, 'Transfeminine Brokenness, Radical Transfeminism'.

3. Alabanza, *None of the Above*.

4. Lugones, *Pilgrimages*, 87–89.

5. We mean everything from carrying heavy chairs as stage manager, which creates a certain physicality and might lead to either new forms of gendering of dysphoria, to the isolation and consistent sitting down that a writing-practice necessitates that also influences us physically and emotionally.

6. 'Ensouled bodymind' combines bodymind and ensouled body. We draw on these terms to position ourselves away from the separation of mind, body and soul. The term bodymind, in the words of Eli Clare, emphasises 'the inextricable relationships between our bodies and minds', alongside the ways in which institutional ideologies – particularly the ideologies of cure levelled at people with disabilities – put the mind above the body, 'defining personhood' and 'separating humans from nonhumans' (*Brilliant Imperfection*, xvi). We consider the bodymind in the context of a world that is already ensouled. Ensoulment means that there are connections to the world that are not based on direct relations, but based on sharing and parallel meanings. For discussion on the term 'ensouled body', see van der Drift 'Nonnormative Ethics: The Ensouled Formation of Trans'; Anzaldúa, *Light in the Dark*; and Aristotle, *De Anima*.

7. Drift, 'Radical Romanticism'.

8. Berlant, *Cruel Optimism*, 1.

9. Raha, 'A Queer Marxist [Trans]Feminism'.

10. Austerity-chic is exemplified in remodeling of public and commercial spaces for an 'industrial' vibe, assuming one has never worked in an industrial space; has comfortable furnishings at home or at work; or *has* a home and workplace.

11. Our thinking on opulence in this book is refracted through Shola von Reinhold's prismatic novel, *LOTE*.

12. Rodríguez, *Sexual Futures*, 104.

13. Nat Raha, in *Queer Capital*, argues that the economic policies and practices of austerity undermine life chances of marginalised and minoritised LGBTQ people, while LGBTQ Rights are proffered as the solution to our social problems. Drift, 'Management and Rights' argues that rights are the complementary branch to managerial control. Rights demand self-subjection to institutions, while managerial control functions more directly as subjugation.

14. Piepzna-Samarasinha, *Care Work*, 136–148.

15. Moten, 'Is Alone Together How It Feels to Be Free? Ummm'.
16. Marston, 'Rogue Femininity', 205.
17. Vergès, *A Decolonial Feminism*.
18. Smith & Stanley, *Captive Genders*.
19. Marston, 'Rogue Femininity', 206–207.
20. Raha, 'Transfeminine Brokenness, Radical Transfeminism'.
21. Holland, *The Erotic Life of Racism*.
22. Vanita, *Love's Rite*.
23. Rodríguez, *Sexual Futures*, 10.
24. Rodríguez, *Sexual Futures*, 13. In late twentieth century USA, such practices were connected to receiving welfare – for a discussion see Roberts, *Killing the Black Body*.
25. See Eng, *The Feeling of Kinship*; Mac and Smith, *Revolting Prostitutes*.
26. For a discussion of this from this period, see Bornstein, *Gender Outlaw*.
27. All power to the trans sex workers making a living through this work.
28. For anglophone zines on trans sexuality, see Bellwether, *Fucking Trans Women, Radical Transfeminism*.
29. To create and maintain a 'Hostile Environment' is the current UK Government policy towards migrants, 'illegal' immigrants in particular. See el-Enany, *(B)ordering Britain*.
30. Prevent is a UK government programme against 'radicalisation', widely criticised for its racist approach.
31. Sanyal, *Memory and Complicity*, 17.
32. Thom, *I Hope We Choose Love*, 113. One of us grew up on a farm and the prospect to return to that life does not lend itself to saturation with romantic queer visions, even if it appeals on occasion. It is certainly helpful to wonder why these dreams are so recognisable.
33. Weinstein, quoted in Puar, *Terrorist Assemblages*, 56.
34. Braidotti, *Nomadic Theory*, 221, comments that 'Becoming free of topos that equates the struggle for identity changes with suffering results in a more adequate self-knowledge [which then] clears the ground for more adequate and sustainable relations to the other who are crucial to the transformative project itself'. See also Chapter 3.
35. Lugones, *Pilgrimages*.
36. Essed and Hoving, *Dutch Racism*; Wekker, *White Innocence*.
37. Rules in organisations function similar to the introduction of cars, which allowed travel to speed up, but also demanded that cities become comprehensible at higher speeds, thus 'sloppiness on the streets' and crowds needed to be curbed, leading to the dissolution of entanglements. See for discussion Sennett, *Flesh and Stone*.
38. See for discussion Weizman, *Hollow Land*, 133ff.

39. Sanyal, *Memory and Complicity*, 10.
40. Thanks to Raju Rage for raising this point.
41. The transformation of a large part of the workforce from working class to middle class in the 1960s enabled a different economy, but also ran the working-class revolution into the ground. As soon as working classes had access to middle class livelihoods solidarity got broken. Similarly, in the UK, the right-to-buy scheme functioned to make working class voters turn to the Tories under the idea that 'property owners' needed conservative politics. While social housing is a great good, the institutions dealing with social housing need not necessarily be idealised.
42. This is partly why we claim the term 'complicity' to think through these matters, rather than Michael Rothberg's (*The Implicated Subject*) 'implicated' – implication implies being a part in a more passive manner, than complicity does. We claim the term complicity because of an interest in agency and how the lives that we aim to form can invite us to act in a way that takes aim at hegemony, rather than merely being submerged with it.
43. Thom, *I Hope We Choose Love*, 20.
44. Lugones, *Pilgrimages*, 140.
45. Harney & Moten, *All Incomplete*.
46. Lugones, *Pilgrimages*, 55.
47. Sullivan, 'Somatechnics'.
48. Raha, 'Transfeminine Brokenness', 632–633.
49. Ferreira da Silva, 'On Difference Without Separability'.
50. Piepzna-Samarasinha, *Care Work*; see also Withers, 'Cracks in my Universe'. Both of these authors are addressing their experiences of collective care among disabled people, who in turn struggle with internalised ableism.
51. Vergès, *A Decolonial Feminism*; Piepzna-Samarasinha, *Care Work*, 32–68; Raha, 'A Queer Marxist [Trans]feminism'.
52. This myth of self-sufficiency is currently alive and well in the UK, where staying free from contracting coronavirus has been deemed a 'personal responsibility', detached from government failures to prevent mass infection alongside decades of underfunding the National Health Service.
53. Marx, *Capital*, Volume 1; Johnson & Lubin, *Futures of Black Radicalism*; Vergès, *A Decolonial Feminism*.
54. Chapman and Withers, *A Violent History of Benevolence*; Dean Spade, *Mutual Aid*, 21–29.
55. Thanking Raju Rage for this point.
56. Piepzna-Samarasinha, *Care Work*, 139.

57. Raha, 'Transfeminine Brokenness', 636–646; 'Queer & Trans Social Reproduction'.
58. Lugones, *Pilgrimages*, 143.
59. Lugones, *Pilgrimages*, 146.
60. Care Collective, *The Care Manifesto*.
61. Chambers-Letson, *After the Party*, 145.
62. Anzaldúa, *Light in the Dark*, 150.
63. Drift, 'Management and Rights', 102. Conversely, one's intuition may be attenuated by one's environment, especially when confronted with repressive institutions or oppressive material conditions (Raha, *Queer Capital*, 197–237).
64. Weheliye, *Habeas Viscus*, 113.
65. Addressing the experience of second generation Black and brown migrants, facing repressive material and social conditions maintained by the state in 1980s Britain, Ambalaver Sivanandan calls a different hunger 'the hunger to retain the freedom, the life-style, the dignity which they have carved out from the stone of their lives'. *A Different Hunger*.
66. Hall, in *A Different Hunger*, x.
67. Lang/Levitsky, 'Our Own Words'.
68. Rimbaud, in Bonney, 'Comets & Barricades'; Ross, *The Emergence of Social Space*; Raha, *Queer Capital*, 55–59.
69. Drift, 'Nonnormative Ethics'.
70. Hayward, 'Spider City Sex', 229, emphasis added.
71. Hayward, 'Spider City Sex'.
72. Chambers-Letson, *After the Party*, 21.
73. Gopal, *Literary Radicalism in India*.
74. https://womenstrike.org.uk/2018/02/01/event-4-bread-and-roses-for-all-and-hormones-too/
75. Muñoz, *Cruising Utopia*, 1.

CHAPTER 2: TRANSFEMINIST ETHICS
AND PRACTICES OF CARE

1. It bears noting that not all trans and queer people experience marginalisation in the same way, or to the same extent. These experiences are lived qualitatively – access to wealth or a disposable income, for instance, may work to protect or alleviate pressures at points, or throughout, one's life, but simultaneously this may function as encouragement to participate in dominant social norms. We have found that

we need to consistently think and act reflexively with our positions and experiences.

2. Care Collective, *The Care Manifesto*, 5.
3. Drift, *Management and Rights*.
4. Valencia, *Gore Capitalism*.
5. Westbrook, *Unlivable Lives*.
6. Piepzna-Samarasinha, *Care Work*, 139.
7. Lugones, 'Playfulness, World-Travelling, and Loving Perception' in *Pilgrimages*: 78–82.
8. Lugones, 'The Coloniality of Gender'.
9. To describe bodies and lives in the flow of norms is to suggest a materialist and non-essentialist approach to being in the norm. Indeed, historically and at present, trans people have faced immense pressure, especially from psychiatrists, to disappear into norms and be stealth about their trans status. But for any marginalised person, being a part of a norm remains predicated on continuing to be respectable on its terms, and not over-emphasising one's difference, and is thus can one's position may be made precarious, including by external forces or pressures.
10. On the politics of the COVID-19 crisis, see Maynard and Simpson, *Rehearsals for Living*.
11. This is grounded in Transformative Justice, but we are also mindful that people who do not *want* to involve the police, do not always draw on this framework (yet).
12. Hennessy, *Fires on the Border*, 127–129; Agathangelou, *Global Political Economy of Sex*; see also Hennessy, *Profit & Pleasure*.
13. The representation of LGBTQ+ workers in the care sector is understudied – there is a need for further qualitative and quantitative research on this subject.
14. Weeks 'Abolition of the family'; Duggan, *The Twilight of Equality*; Roberts, *Killing the Black Body*.
15. Pitt (Cohen) and Monk, '"We Build a Wall Around Our Sanctuaries": Queerness and Precarity'.
16. Vergès, *A Decolonial Feminism*, 75–76.
17. Care Collective, *The Care Manifesto*, 28–29.
18. Chapman & Withers, *Benevolent History of Violence*.
19. Vergès, *A Decolonial Feminism*.
20. Valencia, *Gore Capitalism*.
21. Puar, *Terrorist Assemblages*; Schulman, *The Gentrification of the Mind*; Berlant, *The Queen of America Goes to Washington City*; Berlant, *Cruel Optimism*; Muñoz, *Disidentifications*; Rao, 'Global Homocapitalism'.

22. Agathangelou, Bassichis, & Spira, 'Intimate Investments', 122. The authors follow Julia Sudbury 'to account for affective economies of the diffuse networks of punishment, mass warehousing, and criminalization that come to constitute overlapping carceral landscapes'. They emphasise that this is 'a process of seduction to violence that proceeds through false promises of an end to oppression and pain'.

23. Agathangelou, Bassichis, & Spira, 'Intimate Investments', 122.

24. Ahmed, *Cultural Politics of Emotion*, 45, 63. 'Affect does not reside in an object or sign, but is an effect of the circulation between objects and signs' (45).

25. Ahmed, *Cultural Politics*, 63.

26. Snorton, *Black on Both Sides*; Tourmaline et al., *Trap Door*; Bey, *Black Trans Feminism*; also Simpson, *As We Have Always Done*.

27. Raha, 'Transfeminine Brokenness'; Susan Stryker, 'Homonormativity', 145; Gil-Peterson, *Transmisogyny*. In *None of the Above*, Travis Alabanza narrates the particular vitriol aimed at gender non-conformity, which 'often' includes victim-blaming violence against non-binary people on their failure to conform to the gender binary and 'proper' modes of transness (*None of the Above*, 56).

28. While Hennessy adopts this concept out of Jay Prosser's work, it radically departs from its original source. For critical responses to the problems of Prosser's text, see Crawford about Prosser's defence of the 'wrong body trope' (in Cotten, *Transgender Migrations*, 67), Aizura, in the same volume on the use of travel metaphors (140), and Bhanji (also in Transgender Migrations) on the problem of the suggestion of 'being at home in one's skin' (162).

29. Hennessy, *Fires on the Border*, 126.

30. Hennessy, *Fires on the* Border, 132–144.

31. Da Silva, 'On Difference without Separability'. In Chapter 3, we discuss separability in detail as an overarching structural dynamic of Western, and/or ethnonationalist, nation states.

32. 'Slow death' describes the everyday withering away of life through deprivation and organised abandonment. See Berlant, *Cruel Optimism*; and Raha, 'Transfeminine Brokenness'.

33. These direct, affirmative activities may be contrasted with dynamics of, say, fear, that are primarily discursive, indirect – endeavouring to maintaining distance and produce conditions in which life withers or experiences are negated, fear sometimes animating direct harm.

34. Lewis, *Abolish the Family*, 82–83.

35. Quan, *Become Ungovernable*.

36. On Indigenous practices of care in particular, see Simpson, *As We Have Always Done*; Kimmerer, *Braiding Sweetgrass*.

37. Piepzna-Samarasinha, *Care Work*, 73.
38. O'Brien, *Family Abolition*; Lewis, *Abolish the Family*; Weeks, 'Abolition of the Family'.
39. Toupin, *Wages for Housework*. One of the important lessons from the International Wages for Housework movement is that unequal burden of care labour upon women is a corollary to the unequal distribution of wealth. As part of an anti-war movement, they argued that the money spent on military and defence (in various national contexts) could be redirected into supporting women and their lives.
40. Farris, *In the Name of Women's Rights*.
41. Raha, 'Queer and Trans Social Reproduction'.
42. Piepzna-Samarasinha, *Care Work*, 136.
43. Piepzna-Samarasinha, *Care Work*, 136–148.
44. Withers 'Cracks in my Universe'.
45. Withers, 'Cracks in my Universe'.
46. Piepzna-Samarsinha, *Care Work*, 2018: 46, 47.
47. The 'organized neglect' of the neoliberal state is a formulation from the Care Collective (*Care Manifesto*, 2), who also discuss the importance of making space to hold affective ambivalence around care (27–28). Ruth Wilson Gilmore's 'organized abandonment' indicates a similar social pattern, that emphasises how the prison industrial complex is used to structure such hierarchies.
48. Noddings, *Caring*.
49. Harm is not the same as interrupting activities or feelings or moods. Life is constantly being interrupted; we are held up by a beautiful flower, cat, bird, a talk, an argument, a fight, a book that irritates, by illness, by a broken heart or being newly in love.
50. Stoler, *Duress*: 6.
51. Browne, *Dark Matters*.
52. Thom, *I Hope We Choose Love*; Brown, *We Will Not Cancel Us*.
53. This is the broadly Kantian approach, that relies on adherence to policy and organising oneself as if one reliably maps onto the functioning of the state. See for discussion Drift, *Management and Rights*.
54. Bad Luck is tied crucially to social structures and the material and social resources to overcome it. For discussion see Williams, *Moral Luck*; Nussbaum, *The Fragility of Goodness*.
55. Vergès, *A Decolonial Feminism*, 5.
56. Indeed, we address and use complicity rather than speaking of privilege. Complicity underlines how one acts and restores agency. In contemporary discussion privilege immobilises people by linking structure without linking agency.

57. For a deeper discussion of this anti-static approach, see Drift and Raha, *Trans as Anti-Static Ethics*.

58. This classic example of this formulation is former-UK Prime Minister David Cameron's 'Big Society' approach of the 2010s.

59. Povinelli, *Economies of Abandonment*, 160.

60. Surveillance and attentiveness are forms of an entirely different and unequal nature, where the first holds violence and hierarchy, and the second aims to dissolve these. See: Browne, *Dark Matters*; Beauchamp, *Going Stealth*.

61. Bey, *Anarcho-Blackness*, 85.

62. Drift, *Management and Rights*. Cf. Care Collective.

63. Povinelli, *Economies of Abandonment*.

64. They are what Lauren Berlant called forms of cruel optimism: the focus on what we hope will improve our lives but makes us in actuality worse off.

65. Stryker and Sullivan, 'King's Member'; Pugliese and Stryker, 'The Somatechnics of Race and Whiteness'; Murray and Sullivan, *Somatechnics*; Drift, 'Nonnormative Ethics'.

66. Lugones, 'Coloniality of Gender'.

67. See an insightful critique in Scott, *Two Cheers*, who lays out how educational systems create a sense of entitlement and accomplishment.

68. I am indebted to my friend Jack for extensive discussion of these patterns.

69. Our understanding of navigating the social while practicing consent is indebted to the teachings of our collaborator and friend Joy Mariama Smith.

70. Stengers, 'Experimenting with Refrains'.

71. Kaba, *We Do This*.

72. While social media can be a space of speaking truth to power, sharing information and offering overlooked perspectives, the opposite tendencies of impositions, and speaking-over and machismo are also present, which makes handling nuanced situations difficult.

73. We use 'mixed collectives' here because homogeneity (or purity) is one of the narratives of intuitive connection that is currently available. That there is such a connection can be doubted (Da Silva, 'On Difference'; Lugones, *Pilgrimages*).

74. This section owes much to conversations between Mijke and Jay Bernard on 20 April and 2 May 2023 as part of the *Red Forest* submission to the 2023 Helsinki Biennale: *On the Loss of Energy*.

75. Anzaldúa, *Light in the Dark*, 146.

76. Kaba, *We Do This*, 137.

77. *Red Forest*.

78. James, 'In Pursuit of Revolutionary Love', 259.
79. For instance, people refer to themselves or others with diagnoses, rather than descriptions of behaviour, as if positionality has been overtaken by pathology, e.g. 'they are a narcissist', [and implied is, thus cannot be responsible for their actions].
80. Kaba, *We Do This*, 137.
81. Kaba, *We Do This*, 141.
82. Kaba, *We Do This*, 142.
83. Hayward, 'Spider City Sex', 229.
84. Lang/Levitsky, 'Our Own Words'.
85. Owens, *Love and Rage*.
86. See Rifkin, 'Settler Commons Sense'; Brown, *Emergent Strategy*; Federici, *Caliban and the Witch*; Stengers, 'Experimenting with Refrains'.

CHAPTER 3: 'IT TAKES A NATION OF MANAGERS TO HOLD US BACK'

1. To create and maintain a 'Hostile Environment' is a current UK Government policy toward migrants, refugees, and people seeking asylum.
2. While this chapter was written in the early 2020s before the 2024 General Election, the Labour Party led by Keir Starmer have also indicated that they would take a 'tough on policing' approach to society if or when elected. Abolitionist Futures describe the Labour Manifesto, promising 13000 more police and highlighting the need for more spaces in prisons, as 'legitimis[ing] a punitive agenda' ('General Election 2024 Manifestos'). An anonymous party campaigner described the mindset of Labour Leader's Office as 'benevolent managerialism'. In the words of Michael Savage, 'Labour Party is "Sticking Two Fingers Up" at Working People'.
3. Gender Recognition Act 2004 – the law that allows trans people to change our legal sex on our birth certificates, from F to M or vice versa. The process has typically involved letters from medical experts, who confirm that you are living according to your chosen gender assignment within this binary, and a fee – the cost of which has changed across time, but more recently has been significantly reduced (in part of attempts to affirm the relevance of this bureaucracy). Legal gender recognition in this form is a process distinct from changing one's gender on a passport or driving license (documents that, if you have them, you are more likely to use day-to-day).

4. Gender Recognition Reform (Scotland) Act 2022. This Act was ratified by Scottish Parliament, before being blocked by the Westminster Government, to widespread outcry claiming the UK Government had undermined Scotland's legal autonomy. This in turn has positioned trans people as pawns within the political narrative of Scottish Independence.
5. Wareham, 'Non-Binary People Protected by U.K. Equality Act'.
6. There is a permanent question of how workable such policing in fact is, as it operates on the assumption that trans people can be read as such (or that it is public knowledge that one is trans).
7. See Baars, 'Queer Cases' – we discuss this in brief below.
8. See, for instance, the work of Bent Bars Project, www.bentbarsproject.org/
9. We discuss healthcare extensively in Chapter 4.
10. See, for instance, Samudzi and Anderson, *As Black as Resistance*; Taylor, *How We Get Free*; Escobar, *Pluriversal Politics*; Genova and van der Drift, 'Transfeminism as Anti-Colonial Politics'.
11. Koram, *Uncommon Wealth*; Slaughter, *Human Rights, Inc.*
12. Drift, *Management and Rights amidst Plural Worlds*.
13. This used to be termed 'indefinite leave to remain' in the UK.
14. Michel Foucault and Sylvia Wynter's theories are exemplary for this manner of conceptualising of the binary chaos-order. Liberal-style theories are, for instance, those proposed by John Locke, Immanuel Kant, and to some extent David Hume.
15. To control people by knowing them was the original aim of anthropology. Here again, Foucault's work highlights this perspective, in the phrasing power creates knowledge – yet Foucault does not mention that power creates fields of oversight by remaining ignorant – see, for instance, Said, 'Foucault and the imagination of power' for commentary.
16. Gilroy, *Ain't No Black in the Union Jack*, Chapter 2.
17. Harney and Moten, *The Undercommons*.
18. Bhattacharyya, *Rethinking Racial Capitalism*, 6; Robinson, *Black Marxism*, 26; Da Silva, 'On Difference Without Separability'.
19. Brown, *Emergent Strategy*.
20. Immanuel Kant proposed this division in *What is Enlightenment?* As the means whereby public discourse and institutional functioning operate.
21. The preferred structure of UK activism is to influence officials (MPs, etc.) who propose change, rather than argue for change directly, which reflects this separation.

22. Valencia, 'Tijuana Cuir', 90, quoting Despentes, *Teoría King Kong [King Kong Theory]*.
23. Elsa Dorlin lays out clearly how John Locke's idea of property ownership and self-hood form the core of such a liberal programme, that lead to the violence of colonial forms of life (*Self Defense*, 78ff).
24. Quijano, 'The Coloniality of Power'.
25. Hui, *The Question Concerning Technology in China*.
26. Lugones, *Pilgrimages/Peregrinajes*, 210.
27. At times, it seems that representational politics enter the realm of managers. This is not to say that the structural exclusion of racialized people, women, trans and queer people is not a problem, the problem is that inclusion can simply lead to patriarchy with a new face. It is no historical aberration that members of the oppressed classes are keen to participate in maintaining oppression for either personal gain, ideological commitments, or simply the desire to wield power (cf. McRae, *Mothers of Massive Resistance*).
28. Unions are typically not invested in replacing management and shareholders with syndicates (nowadays). Neoliberal Unions (at best) function to correct management and disrupt exploitative policy.
29. At times it seems that attributing erasure stakes a claim to pluriversal worlding *per se*. However, an ontology that is limited to its own perspective does not seem to 'erase' as such but to impose on itself a single world, which seems to be a function of a moralising ideology, rather than an epistemological action. Erasure seems to require the acknowledgement of multiple worlds, at minimum.
30. Cf. Nash, *Black Feminism Reimagined: After Intersectionality*.
31. Such empowerment without movements comes into being in a very different manner than movement organisers that remain embedded in the movements they are part of. It is only when organisers become disembedded that the problem of overpowered individualism emerges.
32. Kant, *Groundwork of the Metaphysics of Morals*.
33. The inclusion of marginalised people, or of other safeguards of good practice, is often challenged euphemistically, under the guise of 'cutting red tape' to improve the prospects of capitalist accumulation.
34. A regular question in such monitoring is 'if your gender (or sex) is the same as the gender (or sex) you were assigned at birth'. Only the most cissexist institutions ask for one's legal sex.
35. The UK Government's Equalities office, amid government estimates of between 200,000–500,000 trans people in the UK. www.gov.uk/government/news/gender-recognition-certificate-fee-reduced
36. Baars, 'Queer Cases', 17, emphasis in original.

37. Ansara, 'Cisgenderism', 48–49.

38. Ansara, 'Cisgenderism', 51.

39. Ansara, 'Cisgenderism', 51.

40. Cooper et. Al, *Abolishing Legal Sex Status*; Phillips, 'Do We Need a Legal Gender?'. Gender decertification explores the potential impacts of dismantling the legal system of sexgender certification, 'hierarchical structures based on gender and sex, that also encode and institutionalise difference', alongside undoing social injustices and inequalities related to gender and broader dynamics (Cooper et al., *Abolishing Legal Sex Status*, 37). Cooper et al elaborate how such legal changes could have positive social influence, the authors are aware that social inequalities and violence would still need to be addressed through other means.

41. Tasmania is the sole place where gender is optional on birth certificates (Baars, 'Queer Cases', 24).

42. Baars, 'Queer Cases'.

43. Cooper et al., *Abolishing Legal Sex Status*, 17.

44. A 52-page report titled 'The Historical Roots of the Windrush Scandal', written by an unnamed historian and leaked in Spring 2022, that exposes the anti-black racist xenophobia remains not yet 'officially' acknowledged at the time of writing this chapter. A Freedom of Information request of 22 June 2022 has been rebuffed by the Home Office, citing an exemption. www.whatdotheyknow.com/request/historical_roots_of_the_windrush (accessed: 22 July 2022). For a short discussion, see Abbott, 'The Truth is Out'.

45. Da Silva, 'On Difference without Separability'.

46. See also El-Tayeb, *European Others*. In the UK, this xenophobic idea of difference surfaces in, for instance, claims by right-wing politicians that migrants do not – or cannot – understand or adhere to 'British values'. Indeed, the first chapter of the handbook for the British Citizenship Test, introduced in 2013, briefly outlines such values.

47. https://missingmigrants.iom.int/region/mediterranean, accessed 9 April 2024. The conflicts are at times created by European and US military interventions, such as the recurring destabilisation of the MENA region; at times, conflicts are the results of climate change, which is driven by the industrialised nations of the Global North. Barring refugees is part of a wider array of efforts to undermine accountability, responsibility and prevent meaningful action to mitigate or halt disruptions of people's lives.

48. Serano, *Whipping Girl*.

49. One outcome of Brexit is a protracted and devasting labour shortage, resulting from an exodus of migrants from the UK due to xenophobia, racism, and the COVID-19 pandemic.
50. Prevent is a government programme designed to flag up 'radicalisation' in schools – it functions primarily to harass Muslims and other black and brown people, rather than tackle, for instance, white supremacy.
51. Drift, 'Management and Rights amidst Plural Worlds', 108.
52. Raha, 'Limits of Trans Liberalism'.
53. This stands in contrast to transphobic and transmisogynist representation and cultural commentary, which have been simmering since the 1980s, but boiled over after the 'Transgender Tipping Point' in the mid-2010s.
54. For more on neoliberal multiculturalism, see Melamed, *Represent and Destroy*; Ferguson, *The Reorder of Things*, Chapter 7.
55. The 'Transgender Tipping Point' is the title of an article in *Time Magazine*, May 2014, an issue that featured the Black trans woman actor Laverne Cox on the cover. This was understood as a key moment in mainstream cultural representation of trans people, putting black trans women front and centre.
56. Faye, *The Transgender Issue*.
57. Totaljobs, "Trans employee experiences survey: Understanding the trans community in the workplace" (2021). Online at www.totaljobs.com/advice/trans-employee-experiences-survey-2021-research-conducted-by-totaljobs.
58. Stammers, *Social Movements and Human Rights*, 986.
59. Stammers, *Social Movements and Human Rights*, 986.
60. Cf. Spade, *Normal Life*.
61. Gossett, 'Silhouettes of Defiance', 586.
62. Cf. van der Drift, 'Management and Rights amidst Plural Worlds'.
63. Davis, via Marquis Bey, *Black Trans Feminism*, 38.
64. Bey, *Black Trans Feminism*, 38.
65. Táíwò 'Being-in-the-Room-Privilege'.
66. See Quijano, 'The Coloniality of Power'; Lugones, 'The Coloniality of Gender'; Sylvia Wynter, 'Unsettling the Coloniality of Being/Power/Truth/Freedom', and others who discuss the coloniality of power as the mode of regulation of all aspects of life by institutions and categories, each with their attendant hierarchies.
67. Bey, *Black Trans Feminism*, 17.
68. Muñoz, 'The White to be Angry', 83.
69. See Bierria, Caruthers, and Lober, *Abolition Feminisms*, 14.
70. Da Silva, 'On Difference without Separability', 65.

71. Jennifer Nash explains how intersectionality is used in institutions to maintain categorisation and thereby fragmentation of perspectives and solidarities (*Black Feminism Reimagined*).

72. Harney and Moten, *The Undercommons*, 26.

73. For instance, inclusion by means of adding pronouns to email signatures and having toilets as a 'solution' to the exclusion of trans people.

74. One of the lessons of anti-normative theory is that it ignored its complicity in power structures and therefore couldn't acknowledge the forms it created.

75. Bey, *Black Trans Feminism*, 47.

76. Bey, *Black Trans Feminism*, 46.

77. Stryker, My words to Victor Frankenstein: 2; Drift and Raha, 'Radical Transfeminism: Trans as Anti-Static Ethics', 13; Bey, *Black Trans Feminism*, 44.

78. In certain Foucault-oriented work this might take the form of desiring heterotopias that are at the limits of thought to be brought into the centre, rather than a dissolution of a form of thinking as such. These models of thought emphasise ignorance as the basis of duress (in true Enlightenment fashion), rather than domination proper. When domination is unquestioned as structure, it leads to forms of thought that are programmatically pursuing 'the right way to think', which then leads to frictionless thought – instead of embracing plurality and letting go of attempts to gain control over others, whether materially, in thought, or relations.

79. Wekker, *White Innocence*; Essed and Hoving, 'Innocence, Smug Ignorance, Resentment'.

80. Wang, *Carceral Capitalism*. This insight emerges also in Vergès, *A Feminist Theory of Violence*.

81. Stovall, *Liquor Store Theatre*, 2.

82. Or the suggestion that transmisogyny is emotional and therefore individual, see Gil-Peterson, *A Short History*, 9, discussing Kate Manne. We don't hold that emotions or actions are necessarily individual.

83. Essed and Hoving, 'Innocence, Smug Ignorance, Resentment', 11.

84. Abbas, 'Voice Lessons'.

85. Drift, 'Management and Rights'.

86. Raha, 'The Limits of Trans Liberalism'.

87. Care Collective, *Care Manifesto*, 11.

88. Quan, *Become Ungovernable*, 170.

89. Lamble, 'The False Promise of Hate Crime Laws', 1.

90. Lamble, 'The False Promise of Hate Crime Laws', 2.

91. Lamble, 'The False Promise of Hate Crime Laws', 3.

92. Lamble, 'Queer Necropolitics and the Expanding State', 231.

93. Vergès, *A Feminist Theory of Violence*, 9.
94. Cf. Cowen, *The Deadly Life of Logistics.*
95. In the UK, it is illegal to address groups with protected characteristics under the equality law in the workplace, and action to address inequalities in the workplace can only be taken up by individuals.
96. We can see on the other hand, that when structures are addressed by people that receive duress, that this is received as an attack on or a threat to the structure. Freedom of speech is a fight for the power of the white middle class (man) to say what he wants.
97. See, for instance, Vergès' analysis of white feminism's complicity in colonial projects and the institution of slavery, and the defence of these positions by governmental feminists (*A Decolonial Feminism*, 16–42).
98. Cf. Jiménez, 'Spiderweb Anthropologies' and Scott, *Conscripts of Modernity.* Both authors discuss how knowledge can function to keep us trapped in approaches to problems that keep delivering the same 'solution'. Their arguments lean on the insight that it is the framework of thinking (and its methods) we apply that will deliver a result, rather than the content of thought – which is (merely) delivering the details of any analysis.
99. Kaba, *We Do This 'Till We Free Us*, 44ff; Thom, *I Hope We Choose Love.*
100. Harney and Moten, *All Incomplete*, 133.
101. See for discussion Dorlin, *Self Defense*, especially Chapter 1.
102. Two recent plays *The Clinic*, Monique Touko (dir.) and *House of Shades*, Blanche McIntyre (dir.) (both Almeida Theatre, London 2022) wrestle with this problem by staging discussions around Black Nigerian Tories and questions of social justice, and white workers from North England turning Tory and severing solidarity links with their community.
103. Moten, A conversation with Fred Moten, 12 February 2018 Woodbine NYC; Bey, *Black Trans Feminism*; Snorton, *Black on Both Sides.*
104. We wish to thank Layal Ftouni for proposing to think through responsibility rather than accountability alone.
105. Anzaldúa, *Light in the Dark/Luz En Lo Oscuro*, 143ff.
106. The Nationality and Borders Act 2022 makes it possible to imprison people for 'illegal' entry into the UK, gives less possibilities to appeal asylum rulings, 'measures age scientifically' and introduces heavier punishment to those deemed adult, while claiming to be children. It aims to deter entry for 'criminals' including 'people smugglers'. This means that people who support refugees out of humanitarian concern (for instance, seafarers that save people from drowning at sea) can face imprisonment.

107. Da Silva, 'On Difference without Separability', 57.

108. El-Enany, *(B)ordering Britain*, 2.

109. Koram, *Uncommon Wealth*, 2022.

110. El-Enany, *(B)ordering Britain*, 2.

111. El-Enany, *(B)ordering Britain*, 3–4.

112. El-Enany, *(B)ordering Britain*, 2. While el-Enany's work here is focused on the law of the mainland UK, the colonial dispossession of land and resources is understood historically and would be extendable to colonised territories that remain under the British Crown.

113. El-Enany, *(B)ordering Britain*, 18. For a discussion on the coloniality of the politics of recognition, see Coulthard, *Red Skins, White Masks*.

114. El-Enany, *(B)ordering Britain*, 30.

115. Kohn, *How Forests Think*, Chapter 4, discusses this through the interlacing of forest, the Runa, and spiritual commitments that undergird the predictability of life, including hunting. Muñoz's seminal essay 'The White to be Angry' discusses strategies for inversion of social hierarchies.

116. This is not to say that inclusion does not change *individual's lives* (because it does) or even through that changes the atmosphere and discussion in institutions (because it does). Aesthetics can change the world, because it addresses the sensory domain, and through that offers embodiment/embodied understanding. Yet, by itself it does not allow for worldmaking. See the last part of chapter one for discussion.

117. Lugones, *Pilgrimages/Peregrinajes*, Chapter 5.

118. Harney and Moten, *All Incomplete*, 60.

119. Bey, *Anarcho-Blackness*, 93.

120. Lewis & O'Brien, 'The Fantasy of Family'.

121. Haraway's *Cyborg Manifesto* discusses C³I: command, control, communication, intelligence. The C's in this formula require hierarchy, which changed some form in neopatriarchal structures. Self-control and internalised oppression can be brought under the command entry.

122. Here we can imagine that aesthetics and ethics mutually inform each other, and the sensory and praxis can follow each other along in shifting and plural forms.

123. See, for instance, the 1977 Combahee River Collective statement, that addresses how white women ignore anti-racism in their feminism, and Black men ignore feminism in their anti-racist struggles. It should be noted that the CRC rejects separatism and claims solidarity with progressive Black men (in Taylor, *How We Get Free*, 19, 21).

124. Alexander, in Moten and Harney, *All Incomplete*, 141, 143.

CHAPTER 4: MEDICAL INSTITUTIONS, COLLECTIVE CARE

1. Cf. Cervenak, *Wandering*, 12.
2. Alabanza, *None of the Above*, 184, emphasis added.
3. Drift & Raha, 'Radical Transfeminism: Trans as Anti-Static Ethics', 17.
4. Threadcraft, *Intimate Justice*, 145.
5. On the systematic targeting of children under Stop and Search, see www.vice.com/en/article/wx8vxx/uk-police-force-systematically-targeting-children-with-stop-and-search. For discussions on police violence against trans and gender non-conforming people, see Smith and Stanley, *Captive Genders*.
6. Pearce, *Understanding Trans Health*, Chapter 4. For recent, polyvocal work on trans healthcare in a broad sense, see Erickson-Schroth, *Trans Bodies, Trans Selves*.
7. Pearce, *Understanding Trans Health*, Chapter 4, 7–8.
8. Pearce, *Understanding Trans Health*, Chapter 4, 5, citing Stone, 'The Empire Strikes Back' and Meyerowitz, *How Sex Changed*.
9. For a discussion of pressures of gender norms upon non-binary people in reproductive healthcare settings, see Lowik, '"I Gender Normed as much as I could"'.
10. Meanwhile, transphobes, including transphobic feminists, work to undermine transness and non-binaryness by underlining the 'permanent' character of gender affirming surgeries in general, while emphasising the small minority of people who 'regret' the surgeries that they have had. In their arguments against opening the legal status of gender up to easier self-identification, transphobes, including transphobic feminists claim that it may become too easy to change one's gender 'back and forth', and as something seemingly (bureaucratically, socially) more complicated than changing one's legal name (which in many countries, one is allowed to do with ease as many times as one wishes or needs).
11. The relationship between the state and the clinic is not always clear. In Autumn 2017, trans and non-binary activists from Edinburgh Action for Trans Health and the local area challenged the protocol around gender-affirmative treatment pathways in a public information meeting hosted by NGICINS – National Gender Identity Clinical Network for Scotland, a group of clinicians and other staff working across Scotland's Gender Clinics – in Edinburgh. At the time, staff working at Scottish Gender Clinics claimed that NHS treatment protocols were centrally signed off by the Scottish Government's Health Executive (as healthcare is one of the powers devolved to the Scottish Government), and thus clinicians had a limited say in these proto-

cols. As medical 'experts', for the clinicians to claim they had limited power in the process effectively suggested they were civil servants, rather than psychiatrists.

12. See the various editions of the DSM III and IV.

13. Butler, *Gender Trouble* and *Bodies that Matter*. For a more casual introduction to Butler in their own words, see Big Think, www.youtube.com/watch?v=UD9IOllUR4k

14. See, for instance, Faye, *The Transgender Issue*.

15. See Stone, 'The Empire Strikes Back' – this issue starts way before that.

16. Bey, 'The Transness of Blackness', and later writings. Some trans people have been known to stop focusing too much on 'deeply felt genders'.

17. Schmitt quoted in Etkind, 2023.

18. Preciado, *Testo Junkie*.

19. Gorton & Grubb, 'General, Sexual and Reproductive Health', 269.

20. Gorton & Grubb, 'General, Sexual and Reproductive Health', 269.

21. Gorton and Grubb, 'General, Sexual and Reproductive Health', 269–270.

22. This comment is not so much a comment on the trauma of being denied healthcare (although such trauma can have a lasting impact). More, that the wisdom in trans communities that – while often significantly improving one's life – gender-affirming surgeries don't fix transphobic societies.

23. ICD-11 https://icd.who.int/browse11/l-m/en; WPATH, Standards of Care, version 8, www.wpath.org/soc8

24. TGEU, 'Trans Health Map', https://tgeu.org/trans-health-map-2022/ (accessed 5 June 2023).

25. Cass, *Independent Review*. For commentary and an extensive round-up of responses to the Cass Review, see Ruth Pearce, 'What's Wrong with the Cass Review?' Horton argues that the Cass Review is an example of cis-supremacy, within a healthcare system that lacks accountability to trans communities ('The Cass Review').

26. 'Wait Times', *Gender Construction Kit*, April 2023. https://genderkit.org.uk/resources/wait-times/ (accessed 5 June 2023). Average based on waiting times for the 13 GICs serving adults.

27. https://gic.nhs.uk/appointments/waiting-times/ (accessed 30 August 2023)

28. T. Wright et al., 'Accessing and Utilising Gender-Affirming Healthcare in England and Wales', 2.

29. www.itv.com/news/meridian/2023-10-13/family-of-woman-who-died-awaiting-gender-affirming-care-will-continue-fight

30. https://twitter.com/alicescampaign/status/1620050013094289411; www.itv.com/news/meridian/2023-09-20/health-services-in-transgender-womans-care-underfunded-coroner-says. For a further narrative discussion of these issues, see Fae, *Transition Denied*.

31. www.weexist.co.uk/; https://bhattmurphy.co.uk/files/SRN%20cases/Sophie%20Williams%20Press%20Release%2001.03.23.pdf

32. Drift & Raha, 'Radical Transfeminism: Trans as Anti-Static Ethics', 17.

33. Spade, *Normal Life*.

34. Gleeson & Hoad, 'Gender Identity Communism'.

35. Bent Bars Project, 'Trans Voices on Trans Prison Policy', 12. "Only 4 out of 30 respondents felt that trans and nonbinary people had adequate access to trans-related health care. Of those, one said that she did have access in her current prison, but qualified that this was not consistent across prisons."

36. Bent Bars Project, 'Trans Voices', 12.

37. Bent Bars Project, 'A Prisoner's Guide to Trans Rights'. The authors have supported people who received slower-than-typical treatment.

38. Diaz, 'Trans inmates need access to gender-affirming care'.

39. Stonewall & YouGov, 'LGBT in Britain: Health Report'. See also https://fra.europa.eu/sites/default/files/fra-2014-being-trans-eu-comparative-0_en.pdf for a comparative study about trans experiences in the EU (the UK was part of the EU during this research (Accessed 7 May 2024).

40. In their research on trans people's experiences of navigating Gender Clinics in England and Wales, T. Wright et al. note that 'participants may withhold information [from medical providers] or use body language/mannerisms to assuage provider concerns and reduce the risk of comprising access to care' (2021, 2).

41. Murray, 'Acting on the evidence'. The 2017 National LGBT Survey found that, across its respondent groups, '51% of survey respondents who accessed or tried to access mental health services said they had to wait too long, 27% were worried, anxious, or embarrassed about going and 16% said their GP was not supportive'. See, Brady, www.england.nhs.uk/about/equality/equality-hub/patient-equalities-programme/lgbt-health/.

42. Wright, et al., 'Accessing and Utilising Gender-Affirming Healthcare'.

43. While every person's healthcare matters, the scale of the moral panic in the UK media around the access of trans youth to life-saving and reversable medication is way larger than the less-than-100 people of an estimated 5,000 young people trying to access care through the clinics. https://time.com/6900330/nhs-bans-puberty-blockers-england-clinics/; see also, Hilary Cass, '*Independent Review*'.

44. NHS England, Interim Service Specification, www.england.nhs.uk/wp-content/uploads/2023/06/Interim-service-specification-for-Specialist-Gender-Incongruence-Services-for-Children-and-Young-People.pdf (accessed 13 September 2023).

45. NHS England, Interim Service Specification, Public Consultation Analysis and Summary, April 2023, www.england.nhs.uk/wp-content/uploads/2023/06/Public-consultation-analysis-and-summary-on-the-interim-service-specification-for-Specialist-Gender-Incongruen.pdf; BACP, Memorandum of Understanding, November 2022, www.bacp.co.uk/events-and-resources/ethics-and-standards/mou/. For a substantial critical analysis, see Pearce, 'What's Wrong with the Cass Review?'

46. Gillick competency is defined as a young person's (under the age of 16) capacity to consent to medical treatment, provided they have the intelligence and understanding to what is proposed, and are capable of making up their own mind regarding their decision. *Gillick v West Norfolk and Wisbech AHA* [1985] UK House of Lords, 7 (17 October 1985), www.bailii.org/uk/cases/UKHL/1985/7.html

47. Gendered Intelligence, 'Statement on the new Service Specifications for Youth Gender Identity Services', 16th June 2023. https://genderedintelligence.co.uk/services/publicengagement/servicespec-160623

48. This was part of the original judgement of *Bell v Tavistock* (2021); the ruling was overturned by the Court of Appeal (2021).

49. Annelou de Vries, 2020, cited in Moreton, 'The Appeal in *Bell v Tavistock* and Beyond'.

50. Moreton 2023, citing *Bell v Tavistock* (n3). Cass unfairly equalises claims of detransitioning without reviewing how pressures to conform to binary norms inform shifts in gendering at later stages in life, disregarding generally stated needs for such blockers. Simultaneously, Cass does not feel called to explain *why* it would be a negative to change genders more than once. A further failure of the review is the lack of radial comparison between trans hormones and the (lack of) research to other forms of gendered care, with the (negative side-) effects of contraception a glaring omission that highlights the review's bad social and medical science.

51. Carlile, 'The Experiences of Transgender and Non-Binary Children'. This in turn corroborates with the Children's Right Alliance for England research and North American studies (ibid.); in describing key issues in healthcare for trans children, the CRAE highlight 'waiting times of up to 12 months for a first appointment with a specialist service and lack of knowledge or sensitivity from medical

professionals' and 'medical care being available at the discretion of medical professionals' ('Say it, See it, Change it: Submission to the UN Committee on the Rights of the Child from Children in England', 2015, 32. Online at https://crae.org.uk/sites/default/files/uploads/crae_seeit-sayit-changeit_web.pdf (accessed 14 September 2023).

52. Carlile, 'The Experiences of Transgender and Non-Binary Children', 22.

53. Horton, 'It Felt Like They Were Trying to Destabilise Us', 75.

54. Horton, 'It Felt Like They Were Trying to Destabilise Us', 76–77.

55. Horton, 'It Felt Like They Were Trying to Destabilise Us', 77, Horton interviewed 30 parents of socially transitioned trans children in 2020–2021 – 65% of the sample expressed high levels of dissatisfaction with UK gender services (78).

56. Horton, 'It Felt Like They Were Trying to Destabilise Us', 74.

57. Gleeson and Hoad.

58. Research from 2022 conducted by PRePster, the National AIDS Trust, Terrance Higgins Trust, et al, found that, in England, 'two thirds (65%) of people who want to access the HIV prevention drug PrEP (pre-exposure prophylaxis) struggled to do so'. See https://prepster.info/2022/11/new-research-shows-on-going-barriers-to-prep-access-in-england/ (accessed 30 September 2023).

59. Preciado, *Testo Junkie*, 389.

60. Gleeson and Hoad.

61. Some trans and non-binary people do have access to financial resources – we have millionaires and chief executives among us, although the fact of this is a point on which we ought to consider what constitutes community, what are the practices that do (or do not) make it adhere, and who in fact *needs* community for *material* survival.

62. For a discussion of such logics in the case of breast cancer treatment in the US, see Boyer, *The Undying*.

63. Perhaps also a spanner in the story that non-trans audiences are also most eager to hear – listen up!

64. In 2019, provisions in Scotland meant that trans and non-binary people seeking surgeries as part of their transitions we referred to a single healthcare provider, dependent on what surgery they were after: for top surgery commonly undertaken by trans men (bilateral mastectomy and chest reconstruction), you'd be referred to a particular provider in Manchester; for lower surgery often undertaken by trans women (a vaginoplasty, et al.), you'd be referred to this particular private provider in Brighton. This has since changed – although all surgical options for trans women and non-binary people looking to

get lower gender-affirmative surgeries are still based in the South of England – which is pretty far from Scotland.

65. The official name of a 'gender confirmation surgery' is still a bit of a misnomer, hence our use of gender affirmative surgery.

66. Giving this story some kind of ending. Healing takes time, from operations and from deprivations, but healing happens if we attend to it. Collective care helps. There's always going to be swelling and inflammation. New pussies come with new power, different rhythms and energies, physical and psychological. Relieving a bodymind from distress opens space think, act, and create anew, bringing different knowledge and sensations to the surface.

67. Simpson 'As We Have Always Done'; Lugones, 'Coloniality of Gender'; also the denial of gender to Black people who were enslaved (Snorton, *Black on Both Sides*).

68. Snorton, *Black on Both Sides*, Chapter 2.

69. Aizura, *Mobile Subjects*, including on Jan Morris; on the subject of privileging white people in mid-century trans healthcare at the UCLA clinic, see also Joynt, *Framing Agnes*.

70. For example, Jacques, *Trans* and Fae's *Transition Denied*.

71. British Medical Association, 'Outsourced and Undermined'; Pollock, 'Thanks to Outsourcing, England's Test and Trace System is in Chaos'.

72. Koram, *Uncommon Wealth*.

73. For instance, the partition of India by Britain in August 1947, which drew the borders of India and Pakistan, founding them as modern nation-states, took place less than a year before the inauguration of the NHS. Inter-communal violence during partition lead to the deaths of an estimate of between 200,000 and 2 million people between 1947–1948; furthermore, earlier in the decade, famine had claimed the lives of around 3 million people in Bengal, a famine often considered to have been engineered by the British Government. This was a period where the British Government considered the people it had colonised disposable to service capitalist accumulation and war – we were of use when Britain needed labour, disposable when there were seemingly no jobs, or food, or land.

74. BMA, *A Missed Opportunity*, 3.

75. 'Staff surveys continue to show ethnic minority staff having a more negative experience and lower confidence in organisations providing equal opportunities (in 2020 16.7% of ethnic minority staff compared to 6.2% of white staff reported experiencing discrimination at work for a manager, team leader or other colleague). All of which provide evidence that the NHS is structurally racist' (ibid., 4).

76. Shannon, et al., 'Intersectional Insights into Racism and Health', 2131.

77. Shannon et al., 'Intersectional Insights into Racism and Health' 2133.
78. www.theguardian.com/society/2023/jul/01/revealed-record-170000-staff-leave-nhs-in-england-as-stress-and-workload-take-toll. Of 169,512 members of staff who quit the NHS, 27,546 cited their reason as work–life balance, and 24,143 had reached retirement age.
79. For one guide at addressing such problems, see Choudrey, *Supporting Trans People of Colour*.
80. Daoud, in Hassan, *Saving Our Own Lives*, 122 (italics mine).
81. da Silva, *Towards a Black Feminist Poethics*; and Cervenak, *Wandering*, 5.
82. Daoud, in Hassan, *Saving Our Own Lives*, 122.
83. For instance, in the Netherlands between 1985 and 2014. The State of the Netherlands issued a formal apology in 2022, after a collective of trans and intersex people, led by Willemijn van Kempen threatened to take the state to court for a transgression of human rights. The RICH working group at Radboud University is researching the impacts, and Stichting Curatim is producing a documentary about this topic.
84. Tourmaline, in Hassan, *Saving our Own Lives*, xvii.
85. Hassan, *Saving our Own Lives*, 29. You can read the full definition there, which has a much broader than medical approaches and emphasises fighting against racism. Not mentioning it is not erasure – it's a barely disguised strategy to get you to read Hassan's book.
86. Hassan, *Saving Our Own Lives*, 21.
87. Alabanza, *None of the Above*, 185.
88. This includes the 'right' to make one's own mistakes. How else is one to learn or to experience a sense of responsibility, and with that the possibility to imagine other worlds? Stripping away meaningful deliberation depletes the imagination and withers pondering real options to overblown fantasies. Sometimes imaginations need to be rehearsed and practiced before they can come into being in one's political actions. Art is one field where this happens. See the excellent *Freedom Dreams* by Robin D. G. Kelley.
89. Kant, *Practical Philosophy*, especially the *Groundwork of the Metaphysics of Morals*, 4:401ff.
90. Daoud, in Hassan, *Saving Our Own Lives*, 28.
91. Edinburgh Action for Trans Health, 'Trans Health Manifesto'; Preciado, *Testo Junkie*.
92. Kaba in Hassan, *Saving our Own Lives*, 310.
93. For a discussion of trans contributions to abortion rights struggles in Argentina, see Fernández Romero, ' "We Can Conceive Another History"'.

94. For a practical manual on trans-inclusive abortion access, see Lowik, 'Trans-Inclusive Abortion Care', and their website www.ajlowik.com/transinclusive-abortion (accessed 30th June 2024); for a discussion, see Weerawardhana, 'Reproductive rights and trans rights'.

95. See the work of Shatema Threadcraft or Arline T. Geronimus – while Geronimus' work is older, the racism in reproductive care emerges in repetitive cycles. See Thomas, 'Stark Disparities'.

96. For a discussion of these issues, see Riggs et al., 'Men, trans/masculine, and non-binary people negotiating conception'; and Kirczenow MacDonald et al., 'Disrupting the norms'.

CHAPTER 5: ABOLITIONIST TRANSFEMINIST FUTURES: SOLIDARITY, GENEROSITY AND LOVE

1. Hartman, *Wayward Lives, Beautiful Experiments*.

2. This includes not ceding the control of our bodyminds to the state or the institutions through which we may need to access treatments or a means of subsistence.

3. Olufemi, *Experiments in Imagining Otherwise*, 7.

4. *Atelier IV Manifesto*, 12 June 2017, cited in Vergès, *A Decolonial Feminism*, 83. Thanks to Fabiana ex-Souza for sharing an English translation of the manifesto with the authors.

5. For instance, how others identify me, which is perhaps static.

6. See, for instance, Escobar, *Designs for the Pluriverse*.

7. Escobar, *Designs for the Pluriverse*, 4.

8. See, for instance, Warner, *Fear of a Queer Planet*, and in first generation trans studies Stryker, *My Words to Victor Frankenstein* or Stone, *The Empire Strikes Back*.

9. Quinn, in Darragh, 'John Lennon's Dead', 164.

10. Quan, *Become Ungovernable*, 166.

11. In that sense it is the opposite of approaches that look for a reality, behind the reality, and try to 'unmask' others or the world.

12. Overtly prescriptive directions lead to 'I am right' discussions in collectives, for instance, unions, and stage the outcome as if there is only one right thing to do, rather than supporting a reliance on various modes of resistance without the need for a single 'perfect' strategy.

13. Lugones, *Pilgrimages*, 77ff; Bey, *Anarcho-Blackness*. There are also forms of generosity that remain closed – from free gifts by corporations to other forms of generosity that intend to manipulate.

14. For example, rights are 'simply' demanded and granted, maybe while the labour of activists and the people who lived without a pause for

each other, and without a mind for parliamentary representation, disappear. For one such discussion, see Ferguson, *One Dimensional Queer*.

15. Piepzna-Samarasinha, *Care Work*.
16. Vergès, *A Decolonial Feminism*.
17. A lucid scene in Lizzie Borden's *Born in Flames* stages a discussion between white feminist members of the (imaginary) ruling Socialist Party and their party secretary, who demands that they put the needs of the party before their feminist activism and in effect stop their feminist work. In the scene the party officials themselves are not willing to give up any of their power or direction. The scene resonates, because it is so often repeated in struggles, where certain approaches are staged as details to a larger whole. This can be anything from labour precarity to anti-racist action. In familial scenes the willingness to compromise by feminised members, has been classically exploited by patriarchal members to get their way, or care without 'overhead', so to say.
18. See Quan's discussion of the myth of white autarky in *Become Ungovernable*, 24–48.
19. Again, contra institutional approaches, where policy and protocols end up replacing the learning process.
20. Sharpe, *In the Wake*, 102–134.
21. Snorton, *Black on Both Sides*; Bey, *Black Trans Feminism*.
22. Where too often a view of 'womanhood' is reductively bourgeois, centres feminine fragility, reproduction, and care for the nuclear family. Fit trans women in that picture, if you can.
23. Stanley *Atmospheres of Violence*; Raha, 'Queer and Trans Social Reproduction'.
24. Drift and Raha, 'Radical Transfeminism: Trans as Anti-Static Ethics'; Drift, 'Nonnormative Ethics'.
25. In these hopeful remarks, we have to recall the pressures that were discussed in Chapter 3 – where shifts in institutions do take a lot of pressure because at the same time that social change is asked for (or a morality play) the pressures to retain hierarchies interrupt any meaningful change to the detriment of racialised and other marginalised participants in institutions.
26. Hawhee, *Bodily Arts*; Singh, *Unthinking Mastery*.
27. A classic move in, for instance, union organising and centrist to left mainstream politics.
28. We're not entirely sure this is a generational thing. This is not 'leaning in' but 'showing up'.

29. Cf. Mignolo, *The Darker Side of Western Modernity*, 203; Hawhee, *Bodily Arts*, 70.

30. Here we explicitly mean also left-wing management, see Chapter 3 for discussion.

31. Lugones, *Pilgrimages*, Chapter 2 and Chapter 5.

32. Escobar, *Designs for the Pluriverse*, 165–201.

33. Gilmore, *Abolition Geography*, 420ff, Anzaldúa, *Borderlands/La Frontera*.

34. Hennessy, *Profit and Pleasure*.

35. Gilmore, *Abolition Geography*, 442.

36. Gilmore, *Abolition Geography*, 440.

37. Lugones, *Pilgrimages*, 121ff.

38. Darragh, '*John Lennon is Dead*', 164.

39. Gilmore, Abolition Geography, 429.

40. Zurn and Shankar, *Curiosity Studies*, xi.

41. Lieke Marsman is a good example, in *Het Tegenovergestelde van een Mens*.

42. Keating 'Forging El Mundo Zurdo', 519.

43. We do not mean solution-based approaches, or 'easy wins'. Cf. Escobar, *Designs for the Pluriverse*; Gilmore, *Abolition Geography*, 441.

44. By the Hostile Environment as policy, and racial capitalism both as structure and as dynamic we reinscribe – see Chapter 3.

45. At this point it is helpful to read Anzaldúa's (*Light in the Dark*, 146) remarks about how such attitudes are not limited to people with privilege.

46. See de Oliveira, *Hospicing Modernity*.

47. The 2022 London ICA exhibition 'Decriminalised Futures', which emerged from the 2019 conference in London took this further and curated works that mattered to sex work and decriminalisation, rather than have a 'made by sex workers only' approach. SWARM's 2018 conference in Glasgow was also a powerful example of the approaches discussed in the text.

48. Harney and Moten, *All Incomplete*, 57.

49. Camp, *Closer to Freedom*, 2.

50. INCITE!, *The Revolution Will Not Be Funded*.

51. Subar, *When to Talk and When to Fight*, 3.

52. Akomfrah, *The Stuart Hall Project*.

53. As emerging from our discussions in Chapter 3, in contrast to the movement approaches, the managerial model suggests that clashes are only obstructions, which in a sense they are. As a hierarchical model, managerialism expects obedience, a horizontal model of connection should expect and embrace friction because the points of

friction highlight differences of perspective, experience, or ethics, which are the points where a new arrangement can emerge.

54. Kelley, 'Internationale Blues'.
55. Hartman, *Wayward Lives*, 227.
56. Nash, *Black Feminism Reimagined*, 104ff.
57. Williams, 'Why are Trans Rights in Prisons so Rarely Defended?'
58. For instance, the excellent *Mothers of Massive Resistance* by Elizabeth Gillespie McRae.
59. Which also targets non-binary folks. See van der Drift, in *Love Spells and Rituals for Another World*.
60. For a detailed discussion of this on the subject of sex work, see Mac and Smith, *Revolting Prostitutes*.
61. Lara, 'There is Another Way', 140.
62. Lara, 'There is Another Way', 140.
63. Bierria, 'Against Inevitability', 366.
64. These climatic conditions vary according to work, race, and class, and where one is on the globe. For a discussion of transfemicide in Mexico, see Sayak Valencia and Olga Arnaiz Zhuravleva, 'Necropolitics'.
65. Lara, 'There is Another Way', 143.
66. Lara, 'There is Another Way', 147.
67. Hassan, *Saving Our Own Lives*.
68. The suffocating social structure of the middle-classes is partly the result of enforcing interactions that aim to constrict and expel harm before it occurs. In this way whole new forms of damage are created and ignored. This is not to make a plea for harm – but acquiring bruises in a safe environment (for instance, training sessions) can be one way to avoid greater harm.
69. This is not about trauma reactions, but about bodily responses that are sometimes ignored, but influence activity. See for discussion Serres, *Variations on the Body*, 36.
70. Subar, *When to Talk*, 26.
71. Freeman, *The Tyranny of Structurelessness*.
72. Nash, *Black Feminism Reimagined*; see also Quan, *Become Ungovernable*.
73. Julietta Singh offers that legacies are not *the same* structures, but legacies that are inalienable from the previous structures (*Unthinking Mastery*, 66).
74. James, *Seeking the Beloved Community*, 218, 220.
75. Kaba, *We Do This*, 140.
76. Mignolo, *The Darker Side of Western Modernity*, 80.
77. The resource www.revolutionarypapers.org makes journals from anti-colonial struggles accessible and explains their contents in

context. It is exciting to see how struggles draw connections between various sites of struggle that would not withstand academic disciplinary scrutiny, but were very relevant at the time.

78. See de Oliveira, *Hospicing Modernity* for further discussion on our own role.

79. See Alcoff, 'The Problem of Speaking for Others'.

80. Quan, *Become Ungovernable*, 162.

81. Thom, *I Hope We Choose Love*, 149.

82. Raha, 'Queer and Trans Social Reproduction'.

83. Raha, 'Transfeminine Brokenness'.

84. Nash, *Black Feminism Reimagined*, 116.

85. Nash, *Black Feminism Reimagined*, 116–117.

86. Nash, *Black Feminism Reimagined*, 116-117.

87. On June Jordan's 'Where is the love?', Nash, 'Practicing Love', 15.

88. Nash, 'Practicing Love', 3.

89. Insert all of your favourite iconic black lesbian, and t4t, power couples past and present here.

90. Lorde, 'The Master's Tools Will Never', 159.

91. Re: Sonu Bedi.

92. Cf. the writing of Leo Bersani on 'radical sameness' as a mode of sexual desire in *Homos*. This is not to overdetermine talking points such as, for instance, is the turn towards t4t relationality a 'symptom' of 'the cis' having failed us? Cue Rihanna, *We found love in a hopeless place*. But it is to question the conditions that undergird division (separability) and intentional separatism.

93. 'black feminist love-politics asks how affective communities can themselves be a site of redress' (Nash, 'Practicising Love', 15).

94. Thom, *I Hope We Choose Love*, 11, 91.

95. Redmond, in *Making Abolitionist Worlds*, 28.

96. Lugones, *Pilgrimages*, 46.

97. Singh, *Unthinking Mastery*, 63.

98. Hawhee, *Bodily Arts*, 70.

99. Lugones, *Pilgrimages*.

100. Keating, 'Forging El Mundo Zurdo, 522.

101. See, for instance, Karen Barad's work on resonance of atoms and non-locality.

102. Gilmore, in Quan, *Become Ungovernable*, 177.

103. The commodification of identity under the neoliberal form of multiculturalism, where (intimacy with) identities are flagged up as proof of inclusivity, knowledge or social capital, increases this heightened sense of alienation.

104. Here, some hesitation about autonomy (or self-determination) comes in. To be able to determine (for oneself or even collectively) requires a power that sets one apart, from those that are not oneself or 'us', as well as from the environment one finds oneself in. This is not a judgement about communities or peoples that use this term, especially in anti-colonial struggles. However, this book is written in the UK (mostly) with an eye on our situatedness in the continent of Europe. Autonomy or self-determination brings a lineage of statism and being a subject (in a monarchy), which is profoundly unhelpful for thinking a future freed from the bastion of the city state and its Kantian follow up – as we discuss in Chapter 4.
105. Street & Willis, *Revolution is Love*, 211.
106. Street & Willis, *Revolution is Love*, 211.
107. Street & Willis, *Revolution is Love*, 212.
108. Alabanza, *None of the Above*, 188.
109. Lebien, *Gender Fail Reader #4*, 141.
110. With thanks as ever to Raju Rage; see Haritaworn, *Queer Lovers and Hateful Others*.
111. Alabanza, *None of the Above*, 189.
112. We are forever grateful and indebted to the work of José Esteban Muñoz on futurity – even if our proposal is of a different kind. Muñoz provided us hope when we needed it.
113. Muñoz, *The White to be Angry*, 84.
114. Quan, *Become Ungovernable*, 178.
115. Bornstein, *Gender* Outlaw; Wilchins, *Read my Lips*; Feinberg, *Trans Liberation*; Califia, *Sex Changes*.
116. Hartman, *Wayward Lives*, 228.
117. For an introduction, see Espineira and Bourcier, 'Transfeminism: Something Else, Somewhere Else'.
118. This idea has clearly settled in Hispanic theories, yet needs to find its footing in Anglophone theory.
119. Wang, *Carceral Capitalism*, 317.
120. Preciado's *Testo Junkie* has long since made clear the role of bodily experimentation at an individual level.
121. Ahsan, *Shy Radicals*.

References

Abbas, Asma, 'Voice Lessons: Suffering and the Liberal Sensorium', *Theory and Event* (2010), 13:2. doi: 10.1353/tae.0.0137

Abbott, Diane, 'The Truth is Out: Britain's Immigration System is Racist, and Always has Been. Now Let's Fix It', *The Guardian*, 30 May 2022. www.theguardian.com/commentisfree/2022/may/30/britain-immigration-system-racist-laws (accessed 22 July 2022).

Abolitionist Futures, 'General Election 2024 Manifestos: More Police & More Prison'. https://abolitionistfutures.com/latest-news/general-election-2024-manifestos-more-police-amp-more-prison (accessed 1 July 2024).

Agathangelou, Anna, Morgan Bassichis, & Tamara Spira, 'Intimate Investments: Homonormativity, Global Lockdown, and Seductions of Empire', *Radical History Review* (2008), 100, 120–144.

Agathangelou, Anna, *The Global Political Economy of Sex: Desire, Violence, and Insecurity in Mediterranean Nation States.* New York: Palgrave Macmillan, 2004.

Ahsan, Hamja, *Shy Radicals: The Antisystemic Politics of the Militant Introvert.* London: Book Works, 2017.

Ahmed, Sara, *Cultural Politics of Emotion.* Durham and London: Duke University Press, 2014.

Aizura, Aren Z., *Mobile Subjects: Transnational Imaginaries of Gender Reassignment.* Durham and London: Duke University Press, 2018.

Akomfrah, John (Dir.), *The Stuart Hall Project.* 2013.

Alabanza, Travis, *None of the Above.* Edinburgh: Canongate, 2022.

Alcoff, Linda Martin, 'The Problem of Speaking for Others', *Cultural Critique* (Winter 1991–1992), 5–32.

Ansara, Y. Gavriel, *Cisgenderism: A Bricolage Approach to Studying the Ideology that Delegitimises People's Own Designations of their Genders and Bodies.* Doctoral Thesis, University of Surrey, 2013.

Anzaldúa, Gloria, *Light in the Dark/Luz en lo Oscuro.* Durham and London: Duke University Press, 2015.

Anzaldúa, Gloria, *Borderlands/La Frontera: The New Mestiza.* San Francisco: Aunt Lute Books, 1987.

Aristotle, *De Anima: Books II and III.* Hamlyn (ed.). Oxford: Clarendon Press, 1968.

REFERENCES

Baars, Grietje, 'Queer Cases Unmake Gendered Law, Or, Fucking Law's Gendering Function', *Australian Feminist Law Journal* (2019), 45:1, 15–62, doi: 10.1080/13200968.2019.1667777

Beauchamp, Toby, *Going Stealth: Transgender Politics and U.S. Surveillance Practices*. Durham and London: Duke University Press, 2019.

Bellwether, Mira, *Fucking Trans Women. Zine* (2010), 0.

Bent Bars Project, 'A Prisoner's Guide to Trans Rights' [2nd Edition], December 2023. www.bentbarsproject.org/news/a-prisoners-guide-to-trans-rights-updated-kfwhk

Bent Bars Project, 'Trans Voices on Trans Prison Policy', October 2022. https://www.bentbarsproject.org/news/report-trans-voices-on-trans-prison-policy

Berlant, Lauren, *Cruel Optimism*. Durham and London: Duke University Press, 2011.

Berlant, Lauren, *The Queen of America Goes to Washington City*. Durham and London: Duke University Press, 1997.

Bey, Marquis, *Black Trans Feminism*. Durham and London: Duke University Press, 2022.

Bey, Marquis, *Anarcho-Blackness: Notes Toward a Black Anarchism*. Chico and Edinburgh: AK Press, 2020.

Bey, Marquis, 'The Transness of Blackness, the Blackness of Transness', *Transgender Studies Quarterly* (2016), 4:2, 275–295.

Bhattacharyya, Gargi, *Rethinking Racial Capitalism: Questions of Reproduction and Survival*. London and New York: Rowman and Littlefield, 2018.

Bierria, Alisa, Jakeya Caruthers, & Brooke Lober (eds), *Abolition Feminisms*, Chicago, Haymarket Books, 2022.

Bierria, Alisia, 'Against Inevitability', *American Quarterly* (June 2023), 75:2, pp. 365–370.

Bonney, Sean. 'Comets and Barricades: Insurrectionary Imagination in Exile', 2014; repr., *Journal of British and Irish Innovative Poetry* (2022), 14:1. doi: 10.16995/bip.9256

Borden, Lizzie (Dir.), *Born in Flames*, 1983.

Bornstein, Kate, *Gender Outlaw*. New York: Vintage Books, 1995.

Boyer, Anne, *The Undying: A Meditation on Modern Illness*. London: Allen Lane, 2019.

Brady, Michael, 'LGBT Health', *NHS England*, www.england.nhs.uk/about/equality/equality-hub/patient-equalities-programme/lgbt-health/ (accessed 28 September 2023).

Braidotti, Rosi, *Nomadic Theory*. New York: Columbia University Press, 2011.

British Medical Association (BMA), 'Outsourced and Undermined: The COVID-19 Windfall for PRIVATE PROVIDERs', 8 September 2020.

www.bma.org.uk/news-and-opinion/outsourced-and-undermined-the-covid-19-windfall-for-private-providers

British Medical Association (BMA), *A Missed Opportunity, BMA response to the Race Report*, 2021. www.bma.org.uk/media/4276/bma-analysis-of-the-race-report-from-the-commission-on-race-and-ethnic-disparities-june-2021.pdf

Brown, Adrienne Maree, *Emergent Strategy*. Chicago and Edinburgh: AK Press, 2017.

Brown, Adrienne Maree, *We Will Not Cancel Us*. Chico, and Edinburgh: AK Press, 2020.

Browne, Simone, *Dark Matters: On the Surveillance of Blackness*. Durham and London: Duke University Press, 2015.

Butler, Judith, 'Berkeley Professor Explains Gender Theory | Judith Butler'. *Big Think*, www.youtube.com/watch?v=UD9IOllUR4k (accessed 2 June 2024.)

Butler, Judith, *Gender Trouble* [10th Anniversary Edition]. London: Routledge, 1997.

Butler, Judith, *Bodies that Matter*. London: Routledge, 1993.

Califia, Pat, *Sex Changes*. San Francisco: Cleis Press, 2003.

Camp, Stephanie M.H., *Closer to Freedom: Enslaved Women and Everyday Resistance in the Plantation South*. Chapel Hill and London: The University of North Carolina Press, 2004.

Care Collective, *The Care Manifesto: The Politics of Interdependence*. London: Verso, 2020.

Carlile, Anna [Matthew], 'The Experiences of Transgender and Non-Binary Children and Young People and their Parents in Healthcare Settings in England, UK: Interviews with Members of a Family Support Group', *International Journal of Transgender Health* (2020), 21:1, 16–32, doi: 10.1080/15532739.2019.1693472

Cass, Hilary, *Independent Review of Gender Identity Services for Children and Young People*, 2024. https://cass.independent-review.uk/home/publications/final-report/ (accessed 22 May 2024).

Cervenak, Sarah Jane, *Wandering*. Durham and London: Duke University Press, 2014.

Chambers-Letson, Joshua, *After the Party: A Manifesto for Queer of Colour Life*. New York: New York University Press, 2018.

Chapman, Chris & A.J. Withers, *A Violent History of Benevolence: Interlocking Oppression in the Moral Economies of Social Working*. Toronto: University of Toronto Press, 2019.

Choudrey, Sabah, *Supporting Trans People of Colour*. London: Jessica Kingsley Publishers, 2022.

Clare, Eli, *Brilliant Imperfection: Grappling with Cure*. Durham and London: Duke University Press, 2017.

Cooper, D., Emerton, R., Grabham, E., Newman, H.J.H., Peel., E., Renz, F., & Smith, J., *Abolishing Legal Sex Status: The Challenge and Consequences of Gender Related Law Reform*. Future of Legal Gender Project. Final Report. King's College London, UK, 2022. www.kcl.ac.uk/law/research/future-of-legal-gender-abolishing-legal-sex-status-full-report.pdf

Corsín Jiménez, Alberto, 'Spiderweb Anthropologies'. In *A World of Many Worlds*, Marisol de la Cadena & Mario Blaser (eds). Durham and London: Duke University Press, 2018, 53–82.

Coulthard, Glen Sean. *Red Skin, White Masks: Rejecting the Colonial Politics of Recognition*. Minneapolis and London: University of Minnesota Press, 2014.

Cotten, Tristan (ed.), *Transgender Migrations*. New York and London: Routledge, 2012.

Cowen, Deborah, *The Deadly Life of Logistics*. Minneapolis and London: University of Minnesota Press, 2014.

Darragh, Síle, *'John Lennon's Dead': Stories of Protest, Hunger Strikes and Resistance*. Belfast: Beyond the Pale Press, 2011/2021.

Diaz, Jaclyn, 'Trans Inmates Need Access to Gender-Affirming Care. Often They Have to Sue to Get It', *NPR*, 25 October 2022. www.npr.org/2022/10/25/1130146647/transgender-inmates-gender-affirming-health-care-lawsuits-prison

Dorlin, Elsa, *Self Defense*. Trans: Kieran Aarons. London: Verso Books, 2022.

Drift, Mijke van der, 'Radical Romanticism, Violent Cuteness and the Destruction of the World'. *Journal of Aesthetics and Culture* (2018), 10:3.

Drift, Mijke van der, 'Nonnormative Ethics: The Ensouled Formation of Trans Bodies', in *The Emergence of Trans*. Ruth Pearce, Igi Moon, & Kat Gupta (ed.). London: Routledge, 2020, 179–191.

Drift, Mijke van der, '*Management and Rights amidst Plural Worlds*', *Journal of Speculative Philosophy* (2021), 35:1, 93–115.

Drift, Mijke van der, 'Generosity Against Duress', in *Love Spells and Rituals for Another World*. Lily Markaki & Caroline Harris (eds). London: Independent Publishing Network, 2021, 35–37.

Drift, Mijke van der & Nat Raha, 'Radical Transfeminism: Trans as Anti-Static Ethics Escaping Neoliberal Encapsulation' in *New Feminist Literary Studies*. Jennifer Cooke (ed.). Cambridge: Cambridge University Press.

Drift, Mijke van der & Nat Raha, '"They Would Plant the Rose Garden Themselves": Femme, Complicity, Solidarity, and the Rewiring of the Sensuous'. *Social Text* (2024), 160:4.

Duggan, Lisa, *The Twilight of Equality*. Boston: Beacon Press, 2002.

Edinburgh Action for Trans Health, 'Trans Health Manifesto', 28 July 2017. https://edinburghath.tumblr.com/post/163521055802/trans-health-manifesto

El-Enany, Nadine, *(B)ordering Britain: Law, Race and Empire*. Manchester: Manchester University Press, 2020.

El-Tayeb, Fatima, *European Others: Queering Ethnicity in Postcolonial Europe*. Minneapolis and London: University of Minnesota Press, 2011.

Eng, David, *The Feeling of Kinship*. Durham and London: Duke University Press, 2010.

Erickson-Schroth, Laura (ed.), *Trans Bodies, Trans Selves: A Resource By and For Transgender Communities* [Second Edition]. New York: Oxford University Press, 2022.

Escobar, Arturo, *Designs for the Pluriverse*. Durham and London: Duke University Press, 2018.

Escobar, Arturo, *Pluriversal Politics*. Durham and London: Duke University Press, 2020.

Espineira, Karine & Sam Bourcier, 'Transfeminism: Something Else, Somewhere Else', *TSQ: Transgender Studies Quarterly* (2016), 3:1–2, 84–94.

Essed, Philomena & Isabel Hoving, 'Innocence, Smug Ignorance, Resentment: An Introduction to Dutch Racism', in *Dutch Racism*, vol. 27, Thamyris/Intersecting: Place, Sex and Race. Amsterdam and New York: Rodopi, 2014.

Etkind, Alexander, *Russia Against Modernity*. Cambridge, and Hoboken: Polity Press, 2023.

Fae, Jane, *Transition Denied*. London: Jessica Kingsley Publishers, 2018.

Farris, Sara R., *In the Name of Women's Rights: The Rise of Femonationalism*. Durham: Duke University Press, 2017.

Faye, Shon, *The Transgender Issue*. London: Allen Lane, 2021.

Federici, Silvia, *Caliban and the Witch: Women, the Body and Primitive Accumulation*. Brooklyn: Autonomedia, 2004/2014.

Feinberg, Leslie, *Trans Liberation: Beyond Pink and Blue*. Boston: Beacon Press, 1998.

Ferguson, Roderick, *One Dimensional Queer*. London: Wiley, 2018.

Ferguson, Roderick, *The Reorder of Things*. Chicago: University of Chicago Press, 2012.

Fernández Romero, F.. '"We Can Conceive Another History": Trans Activism Around Abortion Rights in Argentina', *International Journal of Transgender Health* (2020), 22:1–2, 126–140. doi: 10.1080/26895269.2020.1838391

Freeman, Jo, 'The Tyranny of Structurelessness', 1971. www.jofreeman.com (accessed 1 June 2024).

Gender Construction Kit, 'Wait Times', April 2023. https://genderkit.org.uk/resources/wait-times/ (accessed 5 June 2023).

Genova, Neda & Mijke van der Drift, 'A Conversation on Transfeminism as Anti-Colonial Politics', *Identities: Journal for Politics, Gender, and Culture* (2020), 17:2–3. doi: 10.51151/identities.v17i2-3.453

Geronimus, Arline T., 'What Teen Mothers Know', *Human Nature* (1996), 7:4, 323–352.

Gil-Peterson, Jules, *A Short History of Transmisogyny*. London: Verso Books, 2024.

Gilroy, Paul, *Ain't No Black in the Union Jack*. London: Hutchinson, 1987.

Gilmore, Ruth Wilson, *Abolition Geography: Essays Towards Liberation*. Brenna Bhandar & Alberto Toscano (eds). London and New York: Verso Books, 2022.

Gleeson J. Joanne & J. N. Hoad, 'Gender Identity Communism: A Gay Utopian Examination of Trans Healthcare in Britain', *Salvage* (2020), 7. https://salvage.zone/gender-identity-communism-a-gay-utopian-examination-of-trans-healthcare-in-britain/

Gopal, Priyamvada, *Literary Radicalism in India*. Abingdon: Routledge, 2005.

Gorton, Nick & Hilary Maia Grubb, 'General, Sexual and Reproductive Health', in *Trans Bodies, Trans Selves* [Second Edition]. Oxford: Oxford University Press, 2021.

Gossett, Che, 'Silhouettes of Defiance', in *The Transgender Studies Reader 2*. Susan Stryker & Aren Z. Aizura (eds). New York and London, Routledge, 2013, 580–590.

Haraway, Donna J., 'Cyborg Manifesto', in *Simians, Cyborgs, and Women: The Reinvention of Nature*. London: Free Association Books, 1991, 149–181.

Haritaworn, Jin, *Queer Lovers and Hateful Others*. London: Pluto Press, 2015.

Harney, Stefano & Fred Moten, *All Incomplete*. Colchester, New York, Port Watson: Minor Compositions, 2021.

Harney, Stefano & Fred Moten, *The Undercommons: Fugitive Planning and Black Study*. Brooklyn: Minor Compositions, 2013.

Hartman, Saidiya, *Wayward Lives, Beautiful Experiments*. London: Serpent's Tail, 2019.

Hassan, Shira, *Saving Our Own Lives: A Liberatory Practice of Harm Reduction*. Chicago: Haymarket Books, 2022.

Hayward, Eva, 'Spider City Sex', *Women & Performance: A Journal of Feminist Theory* (2010), 20:3, 225–251.

Hawhee, Debra, *Bodily Arts: Rhetoric and Athletics in Ancient Greece*. Austin: University of Texas Press, 2004.

Hennessy, Rosemary, *Fires on the Border: The Passionate Politics of Labor Organizing on the Mexican Frontera*. Minneapolis and London: University of Minnesota Press, 2013.

Hennessy, Rosemary, *Profit and Pleasure: Sexual Identities and Late Capitalism*. New York: Routledge, 2000.

Holland, Sharon Patricia, *The Erotic Life of Racism*. Durham and London: Duke University Press, 2012.

Horton, Cal, '"It Felt Like They Were Trying to Destabilise Us": Parent Assessment In UK Children's Gender Services', *International Journal of Transgender Health* (2023), 24:1, 70–85.

Horton, Cal, 'The Cass Review: Cis-Supremacy in the UK's Approach to Healthcare for Trans Children', *International Journal of Transgender Health*, 14 March 2024. doi: 10.1080/26895269.2024.2328249

Hui, Yuk, *The Question Concerning Technology in China*. London: Urbanomics, 2016/2018.

INCITE! Women of Color Against Violence, *The Revolution Will Not Be Funded: Beyond the Non-Profit Industrial Complex*. Durham and London: Duke University Press, 2017.

James, Joy, '*In Pursuit of Revolutionary Love' Precarity, Power, Communities*. Brussels: Divided Publishing, 2022.

James, Joy, *Seeking the Beloved Community: A Feminist Race Reader*. Albany: SUNY Press, 2013.

Jacques, Juliet, *Trans: A Memoir*. London, Verso, 2015.

Johnson, Gaye Theresa, & Alex Lubin (eds), *Futures of Black Radicalism*. London: Verso Books, 2017.

Joynt, Chase, (Dir.), *Framing Agnes*, 2022.

Kaba, Mariame, *We Do This 'Till We Free Us: Abolitionist Organizing and Transformative Justice*. Chicago, Illinois: Haymarket Books, 2021.

Kant, Immanuel, 'What is Enlightenment?' In *Practical Philosophy*. Trans: Mary Gregor Cambridge, Cambridge University Press, 1999.

Kant, Immanuel, *Groundwork of the Metaphysics of Morals*, in *Practical Philosophy*. trans: Mary Gregor. Cambridge, Cambridge University Press, 1999.

Kant, Immanuel, *Practical Philosophy*. Trans: Mary Gregor Cambridge, Cambridge University Press, 1999.

Keating, AnaLouisa, 'Forging El Mundo Zurdo: Changing Ourselves, Changing the World', in *This Bridge We Call Home*, Gloria E. Anzaldúa & AnaLouisa Keating (ed.), New York and London: Routledge, 2002.

Kelley, Robin D.G., *Freedom Dreams: The Black Radical Imagination*. Boston: Beacon Press, 2002.

Kelley, Robin DG, 'Internationale Blues: Revolutionary Pessimism and the Politics of Solidarity', Lecture at London School of Economics and Political Science, London, UK, 17 May 2019, www.lse.ac.uk/lse-player?id=4701

Kimmerer, Robin Wall, *Braiding Sweetgrass*. Minneapolis: Milkweed Editions, 2013.

Kirczenow MacDonald, T., M. Walks, M. Biener, & A. Kibbe, 'Disrupting the Norms: Reproduction, Gender Identity, Gender Dysphoria, and Intersectionality'. *International Journal of Transgender Health* (2020), 22:1–2, 18–29. doi: 10.1080/26895269.2020.1848692

Kohn, Eduardo, *How Forests Think*. Berkeley, Los Angeles, and London: University of California Press, 2013.

Koram, Kojo, *Uncommon Wealth: Britain and the Aftermath of Empire*. London: Hachette, 2022.

Lamble, Sarah, 'The False Promise of Hate Crime Laws'. *Abolitionist Futures*, 2021. https://eprints.bbk.ac.uk/id/eprint/43898/1/Lamble-false-promise-hate-crime-laws-final.pdf

Lamble, S. 'Queer Necropolitics and the Expanding Carceral State: Interrogating Sexual Investments in Punishment'. *Law Critique* (2013), 24, 229–253. doi: 10.1007/s10978-013-9125-1

Lang/Levitsky, Rosza Daniel, 'Our Own Words; Fem & Trans, Past & Future', *e-flux*, 17 April 2021. www.e-flux.com/journal/117/387257/our-own-words-fem-trans-past-future/

Lara, Ana-Maurine, 'There is Another Way', in *The Revolution Starts at Home*, Ching-In Chen, Jai Dulani & Leah Lakshmi Piepzna Samarisinha (eds). Chico and Edinburgh: AK Press: 2011/2016.

Lebien, Yvonne, 'Hallucinate (V.)', *Gender Fail Reader #4*. Be Oakley and Yvonne Lebien (eds). Ridgewood: Genderfail, 2022, 130–142.

Lewis, Sophie, *Abolish the Family: A Manifesto for Care and Liberation*. London: Verso, 2022.

Lewis, Sophie & M.E. O'Brien, 'The Fantasy of Family and the Meaning of Family Abolition', *Ordinary Unhappiness Podcast*, 16 March 2024. https://ordinaryunhappiness.buzzsprout.com/2131830/14680001-45-the-fantasy-of-family-and-the-meaning-of-family-abolition-feat-sophie-lewis-and-m-e-o-brien

Lorde, Audre, 'The Master's Tools Will Never Dismantle the Master's House', in *The Audre Lorde Compendium*. London: Pandora, 1996, 158–161.

Lowik, A. J., '"I Gender Normed as Much as I Could": Exploring Nonbinary People's Identity Disclosure and Concealment Strategies in Reproductive Health Care Spaces. *Women's Reproductive Health* (2022), 10:4, 531–549. doi: 10.1080/23293691.2022.2150106

Lowik, A. J., 'Trans-Inclusive Abortion Care: A Manual for Operationalizing Trans-Inclusive Policies and Practices in an Abortion Setting, United

States'. *FQPN, National Abortion Federation*, 2019. www.ajlowik.com/ publications#/transinclusive-abortion (accessed 30th June 2024).

Lugones, María, *Pilgrimages/Peregrinajes: Theorizing Coalition against Multiple Oppressions*. Lanham: Rowman & Littlefield Publishers, 2003.

Lugones, María, 'The Coloniality of Gender', *Worlds and Knowledges Otherwise* (2008), 2, 1–17.

Mac, Juno & Molly Smith, *Revolting Prostitutes*. London: Verso, 2018.

Machado de Oliveira, Vanessa, *Hospicing Modernity: Facing Humanity's Wrongs and the Implications for Social Activism*. Berkeley: North Atlantic Books, 2021.

Marsman, Lieke, *Het Tegenovergestelde van een Mens*. Amsterdam and Antwerpen: Pluim, 2017.

Marston, Elizabeth, 'Rogue Femininity', in *Persistence: All Ways Butch and Femme*. Ivan E. Coyote & Zena Sharman (eds). Vancouver: Arsenal Pulp Press, 2011.

Marx, Karl, *Capital, Volume 1*. Trans: Ben Fowkes. London: Penguin Books, 1990.

Maynard, Robyn & Leanne Betasamosake Simpson, *Rehearsals for Living*. New York: Haymarket Books, 2022.

McRae, Elizabeth Gillespie, *Mothers of Massive Resistance: White Women and the Politics of White Supremacy*. New York: Oxford University Press, 2018.

Melamed, Jodi, *Represent and Destroy*. Minneapolis and London: Minnesota University Press, 2011.

Mignolo, Walter D., *The Darker Side of Western Modernity: Global Futures, Decolonial Options*. Durham and London: Duke University Press, 2011.

Moreton, Kirsty L, 'The appeal in *Bell v Tavistock* and Beyond: Where Are We Now with Trans Children's Treatment for Gender Dysphoria?' *Medical Law Review* (2023), fwad025. doi: 10.1093/medlaw/fwad025

Moten, Fred, 'Is Alone Together How It Feels to Be Free? Ummm', *Interim* (2020), 38:2.

Moten, Fred, 'A Conversation with Fred Moten'. Woodbine, NYC, 12 February 2018. www.youtube.com/watch?v=I6b5N_u7Ebs&t=622s (accessed 1 June 2024).

Muñoz, José Esteban, *Cruising Utopia*. Durham and London: Duke University Press, 2009.

Muñoz, José Esteban, *Disidentifications: Queers of Colour and the Performance of Politics*. Minneapolis and London: University of Minnesota Press, 1999.

Muñoz, José Esteban, 'The White to be Angry' *Social Text* (1997), 52/53, 81–103.

Murray, Richard, 'Acting on the Evidence: Ensuring the NHS Meets the Needs of Trans People', Kings Fund, 2022. www.kingsfund.org.uk/blog/2022/09/acting-evidence-ensuring-nhs-meets-trans-people (accessed 28th September 2023).

Murray, Samantha & Nikki Sullivan (eds), *Somatechnics: Queering the Technologisation of Bodies*. Farnham: Ashgate Publishing, 2012.

Nash, Jennifer, *Black Feminism Reimagined: After Intersectionality*. Durham and London: Duke University Press, 2019.

Nash, Jennifer, 'Practicing Love: Black Feminism, Love Politics and Post-Intersectionality', *Meridians: Feminism, Race, Transnationalism* (2013), 2:2, 1–24.

Nussbaum, Martha, *The Fragility of Goodness: Luck and Ethics in Greek Tragedy and Philosophy*. New York: Cambridge University Press, 1986/2001.

Noddings, Nel, *Caring: A Feminine Approach to Ethics and Moral Education*. University of California Press, 1984.

O'Brien, M. E., *Family Abolition*. London: Pluto Press, 2023.

Olufemi, Lola, *Experiments in Imagining Otherwise*. London: Hajar Press, 2021.

Owens, Lama Rod, *Love and Rage*. Berkeley: North Atlantic Books, 2020.

Pearce, Ruth, *Understanding Trans Health*. Bristol: Policy Press, 2018.

Pearce, Ruth, 'What's Wrong with the Cass Review? A Round-Up of Commentary and Evidence'. https://ruthpearce.net/2024/04/16/whats-wrong-with-the-cass-review-a-round-up-of-commentary-and-evidence/ (accessed 1 June 2024).

Phillips, Anne, 'Do We Need a Legal Gender?' *Legalities* (2023), 3:2, 127–135. doi: 10.3366/legal.2023.0052

Piepzna-Samarasinha, Leah Lakshmi, *Care Work: Dreaming Disability Justice*. Vancouver: Arsenal Pulp Press, 2018.

Pitt, Joni (Naomi Cohen) & Sophie Monk, '"We Build a Wall Around Our Sanctuaries": Queerness and Precarity'. *Novara Media*, 28 August 2016. http://novaramedia.com/2016/08/28/we-build-a-wall-around-our-sanctuaries-queerness-as-precarity/

Pollock, Allyson, 'Thanks to Outsourcing, England's Test and Trace System is in Chaos', *The Guardian*, 31 July 2020. www.theguardian.com/commentisfree/2020/jul/31/outsourcing-england-test-trace-nhs-private

Povinelli, Elizabeth, *Economies of Abandonment*. Durham and London: Duke University Press, 2011.

Preciado, Paul, *Testo Junkie: Sex, Drugs and Biopolitics in the Pharmapornographic Era*. Trans: Bruce Benderson. New York: The Feminist Press, 2013.

Puar, Jasbir, *Terrorist Assemblages*. Durham and London: Duke University Press, 2006.

Pugliese, Joseph & Susan Stryker, 'The Somatechnics of Race and Whiteness', *Social Semiotics* (2009), 19:1, 1–8.

Red Forest, submission to the 2023 Helsinki Biennale, *On the Loss of Energy*. https://redforest.world/

Redmond, Shana L., 'A Family Like Mine', in *Making Abolitionist Worlds*. Abolition Collective (eds). Brooklyn: Common Notions, 2020, 27–28.

Quan, H.L.T., *Become Ungovernable*. London: Pluto Press, 2024.

Quijano, Anibal 'Coloniality of Power and Eurocentrism in Latin America', *Nepantla: Views from the South* (2000), 1:3, 533–580.

Raha, Nat, 'A Queer Marxist [Trans]Feminism: Queer and Trans Social Reproduction', in *Transgender Marxism*, Jules J. Gleeson & Elle O'Rourke (eds). London: Pluto Press, 2021, 85–115.

Raha, Nat, *Queer Capital: Marxism in Queer Theory and Post-1950 Poetics*. PhD Dissertation, University of Sussex, 2018. http://sro.sussex.ac.uk/id/eprint/86259/

Raha, Nat, 'The Limits of Trans Liberalism'. *Verso Blog*, 21 September 2015. www.versobooks.com/en-gb/blogs/news/2245-the-limits-of-trans-liberalism-by-nat-raha

Raha, Nat, 'Transfeminine Brokenness, Radical Transfeminism', *South Atlantic Quarterly* (2017), 116:1, 632–646.

Raha, Nat & Mijke van der Drift (eds). *Radical Transfeminism Zine*. Leith: Socio Distro, 2017.

Rao, Rahul, 'Global Homocapitalism', *Radical Philosophy* (2015), 194, November/December 2015.

Reinhold, Shola von, *LOTE*. London: Jacaranda Books, 2020.

Rifkin, Mark, 'Settler Common Sense', *Settler Colonial Studies* (2013), 3:3–4, 32–340.

Riggs, D. W., C. A. Pfeffer, R. Pearce, S. Hines, & F. R. White, Men, trans/masculine, and non-binary people negotiating conception: Normative resistance and inventive pragmatism. *International Journal of Transgender Health* (2020), 22:1–2, 6–17. doi: 10.1080/15532739.2020.1808554

Roberts, Dorothy, *Killing the Black Body*. New York: Random House, 1997.

Robinson, Cedric. *Black Marxism*. London: The University of North Carolina Press, 1983/2000.

Rodríguez, Juana María, *Sexual Futures: Sexual Futures, Queer Gestures, and Other Latina Longings*. New York and London: New York University Press, 2014.

Rothberg, Michael, *The Implicated Subject: Beyond Victims and Perpetrators*. Stanford: Stanford University Press, 2019.

Ross, Kristin, *The Emergence of Social Space: Rimbaud and the Paris Commune*. London: Verso, 1988.

Said, Edward, 'Foucault and the Imagination of Power', in *Foucault: A Critical Reader*. David Couzens Hoy (ed.). Oxford and New York: Basil Blackwell, 1986.

Samudzi, Zoe & William C. Anderson, *As Black as Resistance*. Chico and Edinburgh: AK Press, 2018.

Sanyal, Debarati, *Memory and Complicity: Migrations of Holocaust Remembrance*. New York: Fordham University Press, 2015.

Savage, Michael 'Labour Party is "Sticking Two Fingers Up" at Working People, Says Unite Boss'. *The Observer*, 30 July 2022. www.theguardian.com/politics/2022/jul/30/labour-party-is-sticking-two-fingers-up-at-working-people-says-unite-boss (accessed 30 July 2022).

Schulman, Sarah. *The Gentrification of the Mind: Witness to a Lost Imagination*. Berkeley, Los Angeles and London: University of California Press, 2013.

Scott, David, *Conscripts of Modernity*. Durham and London: Duke University Press: 2004.

Scott, James, *Two Cheers for Anarchism*. Princeton: Princeton University Press, 2012.

Sennett, Richard, *Flesh and Stone: The City in Western Civilization*. London: Faber and Faber, 1995.

Serano, Julia, *Whipping Girl: A Transsexual Woman on Scapegoating and Femininity*. Emeryville: Seal Press, 2007.

Serres, Michel, *Variations on the Body*. Trans: Randolph Burkes. Minneapolis: Univocal, 2011.

Shannon, Geordan, Rosemary Morgan, Zahra Zeinali, Leanne Brady, Marcia Thereza Couto, Delan Devakumar et al., 'Intersectional Insights Into Racism and Health: Not Just a Question of Identity', *The Lancet* (2022), 400:10368, 2125–2136, 10 December 2022, I: doi: 10.1016/S0140-6736(22)02304-2

Sharpe, Christina, *In the Wake*. Durham and London: Duke University Press, 2016.

da Silva, Denise Ferreira, 'On Difference Without Separability'. *32nd Bienal De São Paulo Art: Incerteza viva* (2016), 57–65.

da Silva, Denise Ferreira, 'Towards a Black feminist Poethics: The Quest(ion) of Blackness towards the End of the World', *The Black Scholar* (2014), 44:2, 81–97.

Simpson, Leanne Betasamosake, *As We Have Always Done: Indigenous Freedom through Radical Resistance*. Minneapolis and London: Minnesota University Press, 2017.

Singh, Julietta, *Unthinking Mastery: Dehumanism and Decolonial Entanglements*. Durham and London: Duke University Press, 2018.

Sivanandan, A., *A Different Hunger*. London: Pluto Press, 1982.

Slaughter, Joseph, *Human Rights, Inc.: The World Novel, Narrative Form, and International Law*. New York: Fordham University Press, 2007.

Smith, Nat & Eric Stanley, eds, *Captive Genders: Trans Embodiment and the Prison Industrial Complex*. Oakland: AK Press, 2011.

Snorton, C. Riley, *Black on Both Sides; A Racial History of Trans Identity*. Minneapolis and London: Minnesota University Press, 2017.

Spade, Dean, *Normal Life: Administrative Violence, Critical Trans Politics and the Limits of the Law*. Boston: South End Press, 2011.

Spade, Dean, *Mutual Aid*. London: Verso, 2020.

Stammers, Neil, 'Social Movements and the Social Construction of Human Rights', *Human Rights Quarterly* (1999), 21:4, 980–1008.

Stanley, Eric A., *Atmospheres of Violence: Structuring Antagonism and the Trans/Queer Ungovernable*. Durham and London: Duke University Press, 2021.

Stengers, Isabelle, 'Experimenting with Refrains: Subjectivity and the Challenge of Escaping Modern Dualism', *Subjectivity* (2008), 22:1, 38–59.

Stoler, Laura Ann, *Duress: Imperial Durabilities in our Times*. Durham and London: Duke University Press, 2016.

Stone, Sandy, 'The Empire Strikes Back: A Posttranssexual Manifesto', in *Body Guards: The Cultural Politics of Gender Ambiguity*, J. Epstein & K. Straub (eds). New York: Routledge, 1991, 280–304.

Stonewall & YouGov, 'LGBT in Britain: Health Report', 2018. www.stonewall.org.uk/system/files/lgbt_in_britain_health.pdf (accessed 28 September 2023).

Stovall, Maya, *Liquor Store Theatre*. Durham and London: Duke University Press, 2020.

Street, Mikelle and Raquel Willis, *Revolution is Love*. New York: Aperture, 2022.

Stryker, Susan, *Transgender History*. Berkeley: Avalon Publishing Group, 2008.

Stryker, Susan, 'Transgender History, Homonormativity, and Disciplinarity'. *Radical History Review* (2008), 100: 145–157.

Stryker, Susan, 'My Words to Victor Frankenstein Above the Village of Charmounix: Performing Transgender Rage' *GLQ: A Journal of Gay and Lesbian Studies* (1994), 1:3, 237–254.

Stryker, Susan & Nikki Sullivan, 'King's Member, Queen's Body: Transsexual Surgery, Self-Demand Amputation and the Somatechnics of Sovereign Power', in *Somatechnics: Queering the Technologisation of*

Bodies. Samantha Murray & Nikki Sullivan (eds). Farnham: Ashgate Publishing, 2009, 49–64.

Subar, Rebecca, *When to Talk and When to Fight*. Oakland: PM Press: 2021.

Sullivan, Nikki, 'Somatechnics', *Transgender Studies Quarterly* (2014), 1:1–2, 187–90.

Táíwò, Olúfemi O., 'Being-in-the-Room-Privilege: Elite Capture and Epistemic Deference', *The Philosopher* (2020), 10, 4.

Taylor, Keeyanga Yamattha (ed.), *How We Get Free: Black Feminism and the Combahee River Collective*. Chicago: Haymarket Books, 2017.

Thom, Kai Cheng, *I Hope We Choose Love: A Trans Girl's Notes from the End of the World*. Vancouver: Arsenal Pulp Press, 2019.

Thomas, Tobi, '"Stark Disparities": Why Black Mothers are More at Risk of Perinatal Mental Illness in England'. *The Guardian*, 6 May 2024 www. theguardian.com/world/article/2024/may/06/stark-disparities-black-mothers-more-risk-perinatal-mental-illness-england (accessed 8 May 2024).

Threadcraft, Shatema, *Intimate Justice*. Oxford: Oxford University Press, 2016.

Toupin, Louise, *Wages for Housework: The History of an International Feminist Movement (1972–1977)*. London: Pluto Press, 2018.

Tourmaline, Eric Stanley, & Johanna Burton, *Trap Door: Trans Cultural Production and the Politics of Visibility*. Cambridge, MA, and London: The MIT Press, 2017.

Valencia, Sayak & Olga Arnaiz Zhuravleva, 'Necropolitics, Postmortem/ Transmortem Politics, and Transfeminisms in the Sexual Economies of Death', *TSQ* (2019), 6:2, 180–193. doi: 10.1215/23289252-7348468

Valencia, Sayak, *Gore Capitalism*. Trans: John Pluecker; Translation editing: Erica Mena. South Pasadena: Semiotext(e), 2017.

Valencia, Sayak, 'Tijuana Cuir', in *Queer Geographies*, Lau, Lasse, Mirene Arsanios, Felipe Zúñiga-González, Mathias Kruger (eds). Roskilde: Museet for Samtidskunst, 2014, 90–95.

Vanita, Ruth, *Love's Rite*. New York: Palgrave Macmillan, 2005.

Vergès, Françoise, *A Decolonial Feminism*. Trans: Ashley Bohrer. London: Pluto Press, 2021.

Vergès, Françoise, *A Feminist Theory of Violence*. Trans: Melissa Thackway. London: Pluto Press, 2022.

Wang, Jackie, *Carceral Capitalism*. Cambridge, MA; London: MIT Press, 2018.

Wareham, Jamie, 'Non-Binary People Protected by U.K. Equality Act, Says Landmark Ruling Against Jaguar Land Rover', *Forbes*, 16 September 2020. www.forbes.com/sites/jamiewareham/2020/09/16/

non-binary-people-protected-by-equality-act-in-landmark-ruling-against-jaguar-land-rover/#766d57da79be

Warner, Michael (ed.), *Fear of a Queer Planet*. Minneapolis and London: Minnesota University Press, 1993.

Weeks, Kathi, 'Abolition of the Family: The Most Infamous Feminist Proposal', *Feminist Theory* (2023), 24:3.

Weerawardhana, Chamindra, 'Reproductive Rights and Trans Rights: Deeply Inconnected yet Too Often Misunderstood?', in *Radical Transfeminism*, Nat Raha and Mijke van der Drift (eds). Leith: Socio Distro, 2017, 31–39.

Weheliye, Alexander G., *Habeas Viscus: Racializing Assemblages, Biopolitics, and Black Feminist Theories of the Human*. Durham and London: Duke University Press, 2014.

Wekker, Gloria, *White Innocence: Paradoxes of Colonialism and Race*. Durham and London: Duke University Press, 2016.

Weizman, Eyal, *Hollow Land: Israel's Architecture of Occupation*. London and New York: Verso, 2017.

Westbrook, Laurel, *Unlivable Lives: Violence and Identity in Transgender Activism*. Oakland: University of California Press, 2021.

Wright, T. et al., 'Accessing and Utilising Gender-Affirming Healthcare in England and Wales: Trans and Non-Binary People's Accounts of Navigating Gender Identity Clinics', *BMC Health Services Research* (2021), 21, 609. doi: 10.1186/s12913-021-06661-4

Wilchins, Riki Ann, *Read my Lips*. Ithaca: Firebrand Books, 1997.

Williams, Bernard, *Moral Luck*. Cambridge: Cambridge University Press, 1981.

Williams, Zoe, 'Why are Trans Rights in Prisons so Rarely Defended?'. *The Guardian*, 1 June 2023. www.theguardian.com/commentisfree/2023/jun/01/trans-rights-prison-rarely-defended (accessed 7 April 2024).

Withers, A.J., 'Cracks in my Universe', in *Rebellious Mourning: The Collective Work of Grief*, Cindy Milstein (ed.). Chico and Edinburgh: AK Press, 2017, 161–181.

Wynter, Sylvia, 'Unsettling the Coloniality of Being/Power/Truth/Freedom: Towards the Human, After Man, Its Overrepresentation – An Argument'. *The New Centennial Review* (2003), 3:3, 257–337.

Zurn, Perry & Arjun Shankar (eds), *Curiosity Studies: A New Ecology of Knowledge*. Minneapolis and London: Minnesota University Press, 2020.

Acknowledgements

This book has been supported by many friends, colleagues, and allies.

Our thinking in particular chapters of the book benefitted from dialogues and in-depth discussions of chapters with Marquis Bey, Raju Rage, and Jay Bernard. Your engaged reading and comments have provided much inspiration.

Arika provided invaluable support towards this project, co-ordinating writing residencies and for cheerleading the development process. Thanks to Barry Esson, Bryony McIntyre for the care. Thanks to the team at Scottish Sculpture Workshop where Michael Hautemulle, Jenny Salmean, Eden Jolly, and Sam Trotman have been great; and to the team at Hospitalfield, especially Cicely Farrar, for hosting us in Spring/Summer 2021.

Feminism Art Maintenance, supported by the Swedish Research Council, also gave key support and discursive space that enabled this work. Nat is grateful for the invitation and support to participate as an artist researcher on the project. Thanks especially to Petra Bauer, and to Frances Stacey and Kirsten Lloyd for organising a collective residency at Cove Park, Scotland – we cherish the memories of dialogues and time with Marina Vishmidt there.

The book has grown through public talks and engagements, we wish to thank Jennifer Nash, Nicole Sansone Ruiz, Tripthi Pillai, Ina Seethaler and Katlin, Alyosxa Tudor, Sophie Chamas, BAK (especially Whitney Stark and Maria Hlavajova), Beyond Radical: Queer Theory in the UK (especially Ben Nichols, Ellie Green, and Sam Solomon), Elio Sea, Lily Markaki, and Andria Nyberg Forsage.

Across the development of the book, Jules Gleeson, Eva Hayward, Ruth Pearce, River Baars, Shuli Branson and Layal Ftouni have offered helpful advice and reflections. We wish to thank Rehana Zaman for the impromptu photo session.

We thank David Shulman, who has been supportive from the very beginning, and the team at Pluto Press.

The ideas discussed and developed in this book have long been influenced by our participation in activist groups and collectives. Nat sends her thanks to qomrades in Edinburgh Action for Trans Health for your work, support and for changing the conversation on trans healthcare. Thanks also to the folks of Mutual Aid Trans Edinburgh. Thank you to everyone who bought together, and also fed, those of us acting in solidarity with Palestine in Edinburgh, Scotland, during the genocide in Gaza, Winter/Spring 2023/2024 – I wouldn't have finished this book without you.

Nat worked on this book during her tenure as a Research Fellow on the *Life Support: Forms of Care in Art and Activism* exhibition project at Glasgow Women's Library, while working at the University of St Andrews (2020–2021). Thank you to Catherine Spencer, Kirsten Lloyd, and Caroline Gausden for your collaborative teamwork; to the GWL Team for hosting us; and to Loa Pour Mizra, Olivia Plender, and Alberta Whittle for dialogues and critical reflections on care amid ongoing empire. Thank you to my colleagues at the Glasgow School of Art – especially to Laura Guy and Nicky Coutts – for supporting my research.

This book was completed during particularly challenging years in Nat's life. My Deepest Thanks to Nish Doshi, Jackqueline Frost, Sarah Golightley, Kim McAleese, Clarissa Parinussa, Rahul Rao, Jackie Wang, Sequoia Barnes, Bella Cuts, Tanya Floaker, Laura Guy, Salòme Honoriò, Raisa Kabir, for dialogues, support, walks, food, and company during these years. A special thank you to Razan Ghazzawi for deep conversations that influenced my reflections in Chapter 5; and to Jules Gleeson for talking through Chapter 4. Thanks to Mijke for holding down the text and deadlines. Thank you Lola Olufemi, Fiona Anderson, Josie Giles, Luca Hedlund, Darcy Leigh, Sophie Lewis, Shamira Meghani, Fred Moten, Mohammed Tonsy, Lisa Williams, Rehana Zaman, and the team at Lighthouse Books, for conversations, books and texts, and dialogues that fed the fire seared into these pages. Much love to Adam Bainbridge and Vqueeram for your virtual and telephonic reflections and words.

Extra cuddles to Angela D and Claude Cahun Snugglesberg for putting up with my work schedule.

Mijke wishes to thank the Kone Foundation and the BAK fellowship that made so much possible. Without my students this book would have grown a lot slower, I wish especially to thank the students at KABK Non-Linear Narrative: Media Theory Lab, and RCA: IN THEORY. At the RCA, many thanks to Matt Lewis, Cecilia Wee, Nathan Francois, Joanne Tatham, Susannah Haslam, Laura Gordon, Kerry Curtis, and also Noushin Pasgar and Eurydice Caldwell. I've received invaluable support and wisdom from Jay Bernard, who has been a constant interlocutor, Neda Genova, Tuna Erdem, Seda Ergul, Claude Nassar, Chryssy Hunter, Joy Mariama Smith – for the choreographies of consent, Erwin Kostense, Eda Sancakdar Onikinci, Vanja Hamzic, Safet HadziMuhamedovic, Mahvish Ahmad, Mira, Daria Solecka, Lalu Ozban, and Ludovic Virtu. Thanks to Nat for the wonderful drives in Scotland. A lot of the work emerges from collectives and educational spaces: thank you to the Trans Collective and Curatim, Willemijn van Kempen, who fought the law and won, Plette ter Veld, belit sag, Niels Schrader, Bojana Mladenovic, Woehoe woongroep, and big up to the Big Ride for Palestine. I wish to thank *Red Forest* for the years of sharing: Diana McCarty, David Muñoz Alcantara, Oleksiy Radinsky. The people who are closest even when at a distance: Wai Ho, Maryam Babur, Jack Porter, Alkisti Theophilou, and Chana Morgenstern – you have my love.

Parts of Chapter 1 and Chapter 3 appear in a different form in Mijke van der Drift & Nat Raha, 'They Would Plant the Rose Garden Themselves' Femme, Complicity, Solidarity, and the Rewiring of the Sensuous. *Social Text* (2024), 160:42, 3, September 2024.

Index

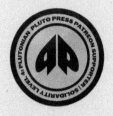

Thanks to our Patreon subscriber:

Ciaran Kane

Who has shown generosity and comradeship in support of our publishing.

Check out the other perks you get by subscribing to our Patreon – visit patreon.com/plutopress.

Subscriptions start from £3 a month.

The Pluto Press Newsletter

Hello friend of Pluto!

Want to stay on top of the best radical books
we publish?

Then sign up to be the first to hear about our
new books, as well as special events,
podcasts and videos.

You'll also get 50% off your first order with us
when you sign up.

Come and join us!

Go to bit.ly/PlutoNewsletter